Current Status and Response to the Global Obesity Pandemic

PROCEEDINGS OF A WORKSHOP

Emily A. Callahan, *Rapporteur*

Roundtable on Obesity Solutions

Food and Nutrition Board

Health and Medicine Division

The National Academies of
SCIENCES · ENGINEERING · MEDICINE

THE NATIONAL ACADEMIES PRESS
Washington, DC
www.nap.edu

THE NATIONAL ACADEMIES PRESS   500 Fifth Street, NW   Washington, DC 20001

This workshop was supported in part by the Academy of Nutrition and Dietetics; Alliance for a Healthier Generation; American Academy of Pediatrics; American College of Sports Medicine; American Council on Exercise; American Heart Association; American Society for Nutrition; Bipartisan Policy Center; Blue Cross Blue Shield of North Carolina Foundation; The California Endowment; ChildObesity180/Tufts University; Chobani; Edelman; General Mills, Inc.; Greater Rochester Health Foundation; HealthPartners, Inc.; The JPB Foundation; Kaiser Permanente; The Kresge Foundation; Mars, Inc.; National Recreation and Park Association; Nemours; Nestlé Nutrition; Novo Nordisk; Obesity Action Coalition; The Obesity Society; Partnership for a Healthier America; Reebok, International; Reinvestment Fund; Robert Wood Johnson Foundation; Salud America!; Weight Watchers International, Inc.; and YMCA of the USA. Any opinions, findings, conclusions, or recommendations expressed in this publication do not necessarily reflect the views of any organization or agency that provided support for the project.

International Standard Book Number-13: 978-0-309-48505-0
International Standard Book Number-10: 0-309-48505-3
Digital Object Identifier: https://doi.org/10.17226/25273

Additional copies of this publication are available from the National Academies Press, 500 Fifth Street, NW, Keck 360, Washington, DC 20001; (800) 624-6242 or (202) 334-3313; http://www.nap.edu.

Copyright 2019 by the National Academy of Sciences. All rights reserved.

Printed in the United States of America

Suggested citation: National Academies of Sciences, Engineering, and Medicine. 2019. *Current status and response to the global obesity pandemic: Proceedings of a workshop*. Washington, DC: The National Academies Press. doi: https://doi.org/10.17226/25273.

The National Academies of
SCIENCES • ENGINEERING • MEDICINE

The **National Academy of Sciences** was established in 1863 by an Act of Congress, signed by President Lincoln, as a private, nongovernmental institution to advise the nation on issues related to science and technology. Members are elected by their peers for outstanding contributions to research. Dr. Marcia McNutt is president.

The **National Academy of Engineering** was established in 1964 under the charter of the National Academy of Sciences to bring the practices of engineering to advising the nation. Members are elected by their peers for extraordinary contributions to engineering. Dr. C. D. Mote, Jr., is president.

The **National Academy of Medicine** (formerly the Institute of Medicine) was established in 1970 under the charter of the National Academy of Sciences to advise the nation on medical and health issues. Members are elected by their peers for distinguished contributions to medicine and health. Dr. Victor J. Dzau is president.

The three Academies work together as the **National Academies of Sciences, Engineering, and Medicine** to provide independent, objective analysis and advice to the nation and conduct other activities to solve complex problems and inform public policy decisions. The National Academies also encourage education and research, recognize outstanding contributions to knowledge, and increase public understanding in matters of science, engineering, and medicine.

Learn more about the National Academies of Sciences, Engineering, and Medicine at **www.nationalacademies.org**.

The National Academies of
SCIENCES • ENGINEERING • MEDICINE

Consensus Study Reports published by the National Academies of Sciences, Engineering, and Medicine document the evidence-based consensus on the study's statement of task by an authoring committee of experts. Reports typically include findings, conclusions, and recommendations based on information gathered by the committee and the committee's deliberations. Each report has been subjected to a rigorous and independent peer-review process and it represents the position of the National Academies on the statement of task.

Proceedings published by the National Academies of Sciences, Engineering, and Medicine chronicle the presentations and discussions at a workshop, symposium, or other event convened by the National Academies. The statements and opinions contained in proceedings are those of the participants and are not endorsed by other participants, the planning committee, or the National Academies.

For information about other products and activities of the National Academies, please visit www.nationalacademies.org/about/whatwedo.

PLANNING COMMITTEE ON CURRENT STATUS AND RESPONSE TO THE GLOBAL OBESITY PANDEMIC[1]

WILLIAM (BILL) H. DIETZ *(Co-Chair)*, Sumner M. Redstone Global Center for Prevention and Wellness, Milken Institute School of Public Health, The George Washington University
CHRISTINA ECONOMOS *(Co-Chair)*, Co-Founder and Director, ChildObesity180; Professor and New Balance Chair in Childhood Nutrition, Friedman School of Nutrition Science and Policy, Tufts University
SHIRIKI KUMANYIKA, Emeritus Professor of Epidemiology, Perelman School of Medicine, University of Pennsylvania; Research Professor, Department of Community Health and Prevention, Drexel Dornsife School of Public Health, Drexel University
TIM LOBSTEIN, Policy Director, World Obesity Federation
RACHEL NUGENT, Vice President for Global Noncommunicable Diseases, RTI International
NANCY ROMAN, President and CEO, Partnership for a Healthier America

Health and Medicine Division Staff

LESLIE J. SIM, Roundtable Director
HEATHER DEL VALLE COOK, Senior Program Officer
ELLE ALEXANDER, Associate Program Officer
AMANDA NGUYEN, Associate Program Officer
MEREDITH YOUNG, Research Assistant
CYPRESS LYNX, Senior Program Assistant

---

[1] The National Academies of Sciences, Engineering, and Medicine's planning committees are solely responsible for organizing the workshop, identifying topics, and choosing speakers. The responsibility for the published Proceedings of a Workshop rests with the workshop rapporteur and the institution.

ROUNDTABLE ON OBESITY SOLUTIONS[1]

BILL PURCELL III (*Chair*), Farmer Purcell White & Lassiter, PLLC, Nashville, Tennessee
RUSSELL R. PATE (*Vice Chair*), University of South Carolina, Columbia
MARY T. STORY (*Vice Chair*), Duke University, Durham, North Carolina
SHARON ADAMS-TAYLOR, The School Superintendents Association, Alexandria, Virginia
KATIE ADAMSON, YMCA of the USA, Washington, DC
ANDREA M. AZUMA, Kaiser Permanente, Oakland, California
CAPT HEIDI MICHELS BLANCK, Centers for Disease Control and Prevention, Atlanta, Georgia
JEANNE BLANKENSHIP, Academy of Nutrition and Dietetics, Washington, DC
DON W. BRADLEY, Duke University, Durham, North Carolina
CEDRIC X. BRYANT, American Council on Exercise, San Diego, California
HEIDI F. BURKE, Greater Rochester Health Foundation, Rochester, New York
DEBBIE I. CHANG, Nemours, Newark, Delaware
JOHN COURTNEY, American Society for Nutrition, Bethesda, Maryland
ANNE DATTILO, Nestlé Nutrition, Florham Park, New Jersey
MERRY DAVIS, Blue Cross and Blue Shield of North Carolina Foundation, Durham, North Carolina
CHRISTINA ECONOMOS, Tufts University, Boston, Massachusetts
IHUOMA ENELI, American Academy of Pediatrics, Columbus, Ohio
JENNIFER FASSBENDER, Reinvestment Fund, Philadelphia, Pennsylvania
GARY FOSTER, Weight Watchers International, New York, New York
DAVID D. FUKUZAWA, The Kresge Foundation, Troy, Michigan
MARJORIE INNOCENT, National Association for the Advancement of Colored People, Baltimore, Maryland
SCOTT I. KAHAN, The George Washington University, Washington, DC
SONIA KIM, Alliance for a Healthier Generation, New York, New York
AMY KULL, Edelman, San Francisco, California
SHIRIKI KUMANYIKA, Drexel University, Philadelphia, Pennsylvania
CATHERINE KWIK-URIBE, Mars, Inc., Germantown, Maryland
THEODORE KYLE, The Obesity Society, Pittsburgh, Pennsylvania
LISEL LOY, Bipartisan Policy Center, Washington, DC

---

[1] The National Academies of Sciences, Engineering, and Medicine's forums and roundtables do not issue, review, or approve individual documents. The responsibility for the published Proceedings of a Workshop rests with the workshop rapporteur and the institution.

KELLIE MAY, National Recreation and Park Association, Ashburn, Virginia
MYETA M. MOON, United Way Worldwide, Alexandria, Virginia
JOSEPH NADGLOWSKI, Obesity Action Coalition, Tampa, Florida
MEGAN NECHANICKY, General Mills, Inc., Minneapolis, Minnesota
BARBARA PICOWER, The JPB Foundation, New York, New York
SUE PECHILIO POLIS, National League of Cities, Washington, DC
ROBERT C. POST, Chobani, New York, New York
AMELIE G. RAMIREZ, Salud America!, San Antonio, Texas
OLIVIA ROANHORSE, Notah Begay III Foundation, Santa Ana Pueblo, New Mexico
NANCY ROMAN, Partnership for a Healthier America, Washington, DC
KEVIN R. RONNEBERG, HealthPartners, Inc., Minneapolis, Minnesota
SYLVIA ROWE, SR Strategy, LLC, Washington, DC
JAMES F. SALLIS, University of California, San Diego
MARION STANDISH, The California Endowment, Oakland, California
KATHLEEN TULLIE, Reebok International, Canton, Massachusetts
MONICA HOBBS VINLUAN, Robert Wood Johnson Foundation, Princeton, New Jersey
JAMES R. WHITEHEAD, American College of Sports Medicine, Indianapolis, Indiana
TRACY ZVENYACH, Novo Nordisk, Washington, DC

Health and Medicine Division Staff

LESLIE J. SIM, Roundtable Director
HEATHER DEL VALLE COOK, Senior Program Officer
ELLE ALEXANDER, Associate Program Officer
AMANDA NGUYEN, Associate Program Officer
MEREDITH YOUNG, Research Assistant
CYPRESS LYNX, Senior Program Assistant
ANN L. YAKTINE, Food and Nutrition Board Director

Consultant

WILLIAM (BILL) H. DIETZ, The George Washington University, Washington, DC

Reviewers

This Proceedings of a Workshop was reviewed in draft form by individuals chosen for their diverse perspectives and technical expertise. The purpose of this independent review is to provide candid and critical comments that will assist the National Academies of Sciences, Engineering, and Medicine in making each published proceedings as sound as possible and to ensure that it meets the institutional standards for quality, objectivity, evidence, and responsiveness to the charge. The review comments and draft manuscript remain confidential to protect the integrity of the process.

We thank the following individuals for their review of this proceedings:

ANNE M. DATTILO, Nestlé Nutrition
JENNIFER FASSBENDER, Reinvestment Fund
CORINNA HAWKES, City, University of London
RACHEL NUGENT, RTI International

Although the reviewers listed above provided many constructive comments and suggestions, they were not asked to endorse the content of the proceedings, nor did they see the final draft before its release. The review of this proceedings was overseen by **CHERYL A. M. ANDERSON,** University of California, San Diego. She was responsible for making certain that an independent examination of this proceedings was carried out in accordance with standards of the National Academies and that all review comments were carefully considered. Responsibility for the final content rests entirely with the rapporteur and the National Academies.

Contents

1 **INTRODUCTION**   1
Introductory Remarks, 1
Organization of This Proceedings, 3

2 **GLOBAL TRENDS IN OBESITY**   5
Global Trends in Body Mass Index and Obesity, 6
Obesity in Asian Populations, 11
Obesity in African Migrant and Nonmigrant Populations, 14
The Double Burden of Malnutrition, 20
Discussion, 24

3 **GLOBAL OBESITY PREVENTION AND TREATMENT EFFORTS**   27
Management and Advocacy for Providers, Patients, and Systems, 28
More Active People for a Healthier World, 30
Food and Nutrition Initiatives in Latin America and the Caribbean, 35
Discussion, 38

4 **MANAGING THE GLOBAL EPIDEMIC: CHALLENGES AND CROSS-CULTURAL INSIGHTS**   41
Navigating the Obesity Epidemic: The Mexico Experience, 42
Common Threads in Obesity Risk Among Racial/Ethnic and Migrant Minority Populations, 45

The Contribution of Traditional Cultures to Resolving the Obesity Pandemic, 48
Discussion, 50

5 REFLECTIONS ON THE GLOBAL APPROACH AND LESSONS FOR NEXT STEPS   53
Global Lessons for Physical Activity Promotion in the United States, 54
Public Policies to Improve the Food Environment, 56
A Perspective from the World Bank, 57
Tying It All Together, 59
Discussion, 60

REFERENCES   63

APPENDIXES
A   WORKSHOP AGENDA   71
B   ACRONYMS AND ABBREVIATIONS   73
C   BIOGRAPHICAL SKETCHES OF WORKSHOP SPEAKERS AND PLANNING COMMITTEE MEMBERS   75

Box, Figures, and Table

BOX

1-1 Workshop Statement of Task, 2

FIGURES

2-1 Global trends in adult body mass index (BMI), 7
2-2 Body mass index (BMI) trends in children and adolescents (aged 5–19 years), 7
2-3 Trends in the global prevalence of obesity, 8
2-4 Trends in global age-standardized prevalence of body mass index (BMI) categories in men and women, 9
2-5 Trends in global age-standardized prevalence of body mass index (BMI) categories in male and female children and adolescents (aged 5–19 years), 10
2-6 Prevalence of obesity (body mass index [BMI] >30) in adults (aged 18+ years) by world region, 11
2-7 Global trends in type 2 diabetes prevalence, 12
2-8 Ghanaians' prevalence of overweight and obesity (body mass index [BMI] ≥25) by age and location, 17
2-9 Ghanaians' age-standardized prevalence of overweight and obesity (body mass index [BMI] ≥25) by locality, 18
2-10 Ghanaians' age-standardized prevalence of type 2 diabetes (World Health Organization criteria) by locality, 19

2-11 Drivers and conditions associated with the double burden: stages of modern agricultural and food system development, 22

3-1 Greatest barriers to obesity treatment, as reported by the World Obesity Federation, 30
3-2 Example of a country report card in the World Obesity Federation's Management Advocacy for Providers, Patients, and Systems (MAPPS) program, 31
3-3 Percentage of people who do not meet physical activity recommendations, by sex and global region, 33
3-4 Percentage of people who do not meet physical activity recommendations, by World Bank income classification, 34

4-1 Warning label system implemented in Chile and Guideline Daily Amount label system implemented in Mexico, 43
4-2 Pathway for production of racial/ethnic and migrant inequities in obesity and potential points to intervene, 48

5-1 Walking for transportation and leisure: differences by race/ethnicity, 54

TABLE

4-1 Potential Influences on Obesity in Minority Populations of Color, 47

1

Introduction

A workshop titled Current Status and Response to the Global Obesity Epidemic, held October 9, 2018, in Washington, DC, was convened by the Roundtable on Obesity Solutions, Health and Medicine Division, National Academies of Sciences, Engineering, and Medicine. The workshop examined the status of the global obesity pandemic[1] and explored approaches used to address the problem in different settings around the world. Invited presenters discussed the importance of understanding the obesity epidemic in a global context and shared perspectives on the implications of this understanding of the problem for prevention and treatment efforts in the United States, with an emphasis on reducing disparities. The workshop's full Statement of Task is in Box 1-1.[2]

INTRODUCTORY REMARKS

Bill Purcell of Farmer Purcell White & Lassiter, PLLC, and chair of the Roundtable on Obesity Solutions, welcomed participants and provided a brief overview of the roundtable. He explained that the roundtable engages leaders from multiple sectors to help solve the nation's obesity

---

[1] The Centers for Disease Control and Prevention (CDC) defines a pandemic as an epidemic that has spread over several countries or continents, usually affecting a large number of people. See https://www.cdc.gov/ophss/csels/dsepd/ss1978/lesson1/section11.html (accessed January 29, 2019).

[2] The workshop agenda, presentations, and other materials are available at http://www.nationalacademies.org/hmd/Activities/Nutrition/ObesitySolutions/2018-OCT-9.aspx (accessed January 29, 2019).

> **BOX 1-1**
> **Workshop Statement of Task**
>
> An ad hoc committee will plan and conduct a 1-day public workshop that will feature invited presentations and discussions to examine the status of the global obesity pandemic and explore approaches aimed at managing the problem in different settings around the world. Workshop presentations will characterize the nature of obesity and discuss the importance of understanding the obesity epidemic in global context. The workshop will also include perspectives on the implications of obesity as a global problem for prevention and treatment efforts in the United States, with an emphasis on reducing disparities. The workshop will explore the current state of the science on prevalence, trends, cost, and drivers of obesity globally, focusing on country or regional differences. Presentations and discussions will highlight efforts to identify, promote, and monitor policy and systems initiatives related to obesity prevention and control—related to nutrition and physical activity—worldwide. Using country- or region-specific examples, discussion will highlight the complexity of the global approach to managing the obesity epidemic (e.g., how it is embedded in the response to addressing non-communicable diseases, the "double burden" of undernutrition and obesity, and implementation challenges in low and middle-income countries).

crisis by preventing and treating obesity and its consequences across the lifespan. Through meetings, public workshops, background papers, and ad hoc convening activities, it fosters an ongoing dialogue about critical and emerging issues in obesity prevention and treatment, he continued. He explained further that the roundtable also provides a trusted venue for inspiring, developing, and examining multisector collaborations as well as policy, environmental, and behavioral initiatives designed to increase physical activity, reduce sedentary behavior, and improve the healthfulness of foods and beverages, with the goal of reducing the prevalence and adverse consequences of obesity and its related health disparities.

Purcell outlined the workshop's four sessions and noted its timeliness, as it occurred during National Obesity Care Week and 2 days prior to World Obesity Day. He closed by telling participants that the roundtable hopes to encourage, enhance, and sustain action for partnerships and collaborations. "Watching you gather here today," he said, "made me believe that this is a group that knows not just this work but each other well, and is collaborating now, and we hope and believe will continue to collaborate and perhaps enhance your collaborations going forward to end this pandemic."

ORGANIZATION OF THIS PROCEEDINGS

This proceedings follows the order of the workshop agenda (see Appendix A), chronicling its four sessions in individual chapters. Chapter 2 explores global trends in obesity and examines its collective prevalence, costs, and drivers around the world, including country and regional differences. Chapter 3 highlights global efforts to identify, promote, and monitor policy and systems initiatives related to obesity prevention and control. Chapter 4 reviews challenges and cross-cultural insights associated with efforts to prevent and control obesity. Finally, Chapter 5 reflects on progress to date and summarizes lessons for prevention and treatment efforts in the United States. Appendix B is a list of acronyms and abbreviations used in this proceedings, while Appendix C presents biographical sketches of the workshop speakers and planning committee members.

2

Global Trends in Obesity

> **Highlights from the Presentations of Individual Speakers**
> - Obesity is increasing in every region of the world, and the overall proportion of adult men and women in the high body mass index (BMI) category (≥ 25 kg/m^2) has now surpassed the proportion in the low BMI category (<20 kg/m^2). Data show that 50 million girls, 74 million boys, 390 million women, and 281 million men worldwide were estimated to have obesity in 2016. (Lindsay Jaacks)
> - Obesity prevalence has increased in Asia over recent decades, but still remains lower than in other world regions. Asians develop diabetes at lower weights, at younger ages, and more rapidly compared with Western populations. Incorporating Asian-specific BMI and waist circumference cutoff points into screening programs could help reduce the burden of chronic disease in this population. (Vasanti Malik)
> - The world is experiencing rapid ethnic diversification due to an increase in international migration, and there is a high burden of overweight and obesity among African migrants in Europe. Assessing migrant health can help unravel the complex interplay between genetic and environmental determinants of obesity. (Karlijn Meeks)
> - The framing of the double burden of malnutrition as "malnutrition in all its forms" is becoming more accepted,

> although many of the relationships between undernutrition and overweight/obesity are not yet fully understood. "Double-duty" interventions that address both forms of malnutrition could be prioritized. (Rachel Nugent)

The first session of the workshop, moderated by Christina Economos, co-founder and director of ChildObesity180 and professor and New Balance chair in childhood nutrition at the Friedman School of Nutrition Science and Policy, Tufts University, described global trends in obesity and examined its collective prevalence, costs, and drivers worldwide while also highlighting country and regional differences.

GLOBAL TRENDS IN BODY MASS INDEX AND OBESITY

Lindsay Jaacks, assistant professor in the Department of Global Health and Population, Harvard T.H. Chan School of Public Health, and visiting professor at the Public Health Foundation of India in Delhi, set the stage for her talk by stating that obesity is increasing in all regions of the world. She began by discussing global trends in body mass index (BMI) and obesity, pointing to contrasts in these trends between adults and children around the world.

Jaacks reported that adult BMI has increased steadily in the United States and worldwide, according to measured height and weight data from the Noncommunicable Diseases Risk Factor Collaboration (NCD-RisC) for 1975 through 2016 (see Figure 2-1). These trends show "no sign of any substantial plateau, let alone a decrease," she commented. She speculated that these trends influenced the World Health Organization's (WHO's) target for overweight and obesity, simply to halt the increase in prevalence rather than achieve a decline.

Jaacks again referenced data from NCD-RisC to highlight a global trend of increasing BMI among children and adolescents (aged 5–19 years). She noted, however, that the rise in BMI in this age group has not been as steep as that among adults (see Figure 2-2). She explained that despite this apparent lag in the prevalence of child and adolescent overweight and obesity, BMI for this age group is still increasing globally, and a plateau or decline has been observed only in certain sociodemographic groups in a handful of countries.

Jaacks went on to discuss regional differences in mean BMI, based on NCD-RisC data. She highlighted large increases in mean BMI in females in South and East Asia, especially among children. She noted that the dataset's East Asia region excluded high-income countries such as Japan and South Korea, which she said have observed a plateau in overweight and obesity

GLOBAL TRENDS IN OBESITY 7

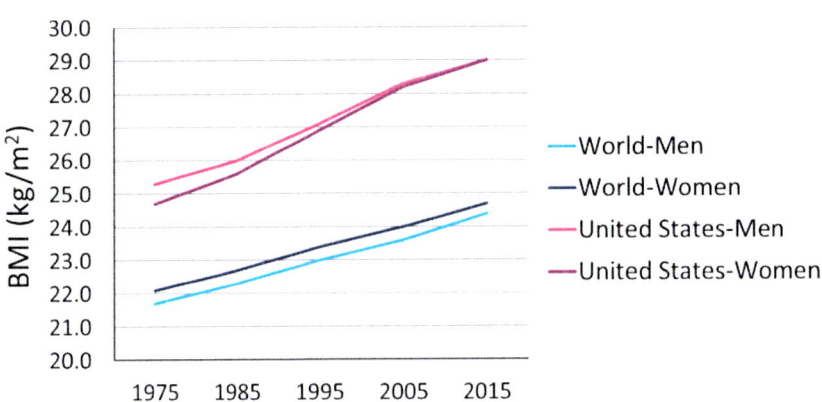

FIGURE 2-1 Global trends in adult body mass index (BMI).
SOURCES: NCD-RisC, 2017. Presented by Lindsay Jaacks, October 9, 2018. Reprinted with permission from Elsevier.

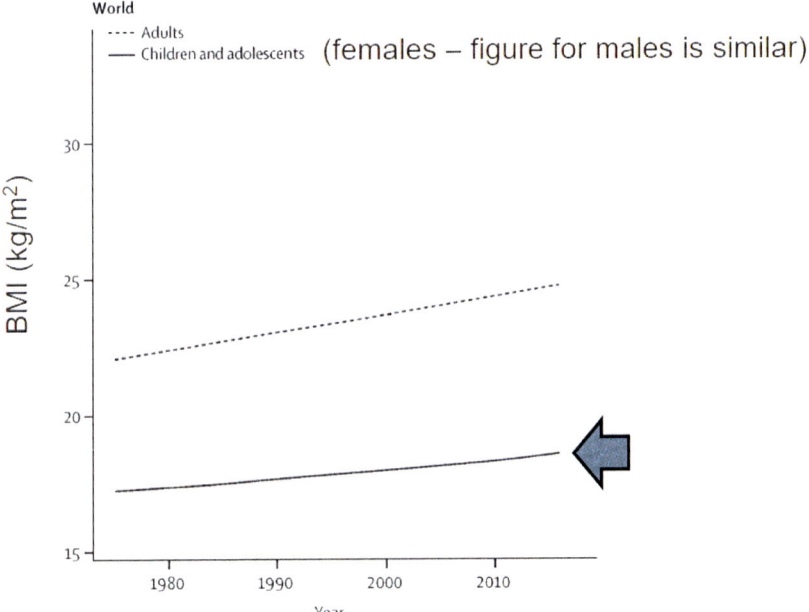

FIGURE 2-2 Body mass index (BMI) trends in children and adolescents (aged 5–19 years).
SOURCES: NCD-RisC, 2017. Presented by Lindsay Jaacks, October 9, 2018. Reprinted with permission from Elsevier.

prevalence among females. For males, she reported, the data show a steady increase in mean BMI in South, Southeast, and East Asia (NCD-RisC, 2017). Given these trends, she suggested, it is not surprising that there are "huge increases" in the prevalence of obesity globally when the binary indicator of BMI is used.

Jaacks illustrated those overall increases by comparing the global prevalence of obesity in 1975 with the most recent estimates for adults and children (see Figure 2-3). She reported that global obesity prevalence has risen approximately 2 percentage points per decade (NCD-RisC, 2016, 2017). When the first estimates of obesity were available in 1975, she remarked, Russia was the only country with a prevalence greater than 5 percent (NCD-RisC, 2017). Now, she continued, about half of the world's most populous countries have a prevalence greater than 20 percent. Since 1975, she summarized, there has been a "remarkable increase" in the prevalence of obesity across almost all countries and in all regions of the world.

Jaacks then displayed world maps illustrating differences in obesity prevalence among countries for men, women, boys, and girls. These maps show that the highest prevalence of obesity globally occurs in Pacific Island countries, where it reaches upwards of 60 percent. Prevalence in this region was high initially, and its increase has been substantial, Jaacks observed, especially relative to high-income Asian countries, such as Japan and South Korea, that have an obesity prevalence of around 5 percent (NCD-RisC, 2016, 2017). She added that countries with lower gross domestic product (GDP) tend to have a higher obesity prevalence among women than among

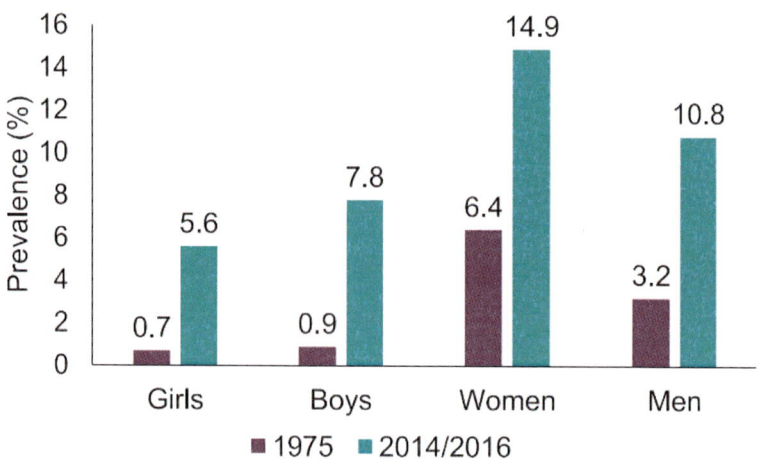

FIGURE 2-3 Trends in the global prevalence of obesity.
SOURCES: NCD-RisC, 2016, 2017. Presented by Lindsay Jaacks, October 9, 2018. Reprinted with permission from Elsevier.

men. As GDP rises, she said, women and men approach each other in obesity prevalence.

Next, Jaacks shared data on the global proportions of adult men and women in low (<20 kg/m^2), normal (20 to <25 kg/m^2), and high (≥25 kg/m^2) BMI categories across several decades. For the first time in history, she remarked, the overall proportion in the high BMI category has surpassed the proportion in the low BMI category for both sexes, according to the most recent data (see Figure 2-4). She acknowledged that globally, undernutrition is still more prevalent than high BMI among children and adolescents (see Figure 2-5), but she cited a projection that the opposite will be true by 2022 if trends of increasing BMI continue (NCD-RisC, 2017).

Jaacks then offered examples of socioeconomic differences, referencing data indicating that women in the top education quartile are more likely to be overweight than those in the bottom quartile, up until a relatively high level of country GDP. Beyond that GDP threshold, she said, women with the least education have a consistently greater probability of being overweight (Goryakin and Suhrcke, 2014). She suggested that this finding helps explain national differences in the prevalence of overweight and

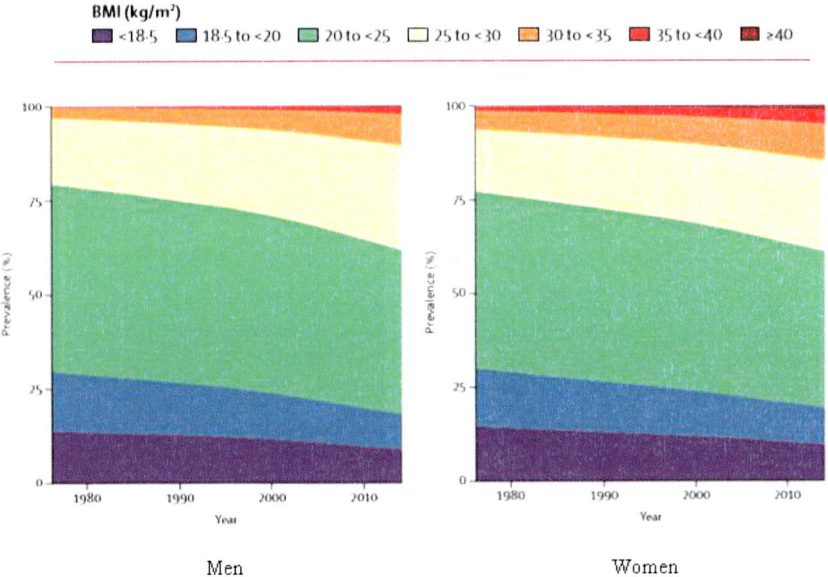

FIGURE 2-4 Trends in global age-standardized prevalence of body mass index (BMI) categories in men and women.
SOURCES: NCD-RisC, 2016. Presented by Lindsay Jaacks, October 9, 2018. Reprinted with permission from Elsevier.

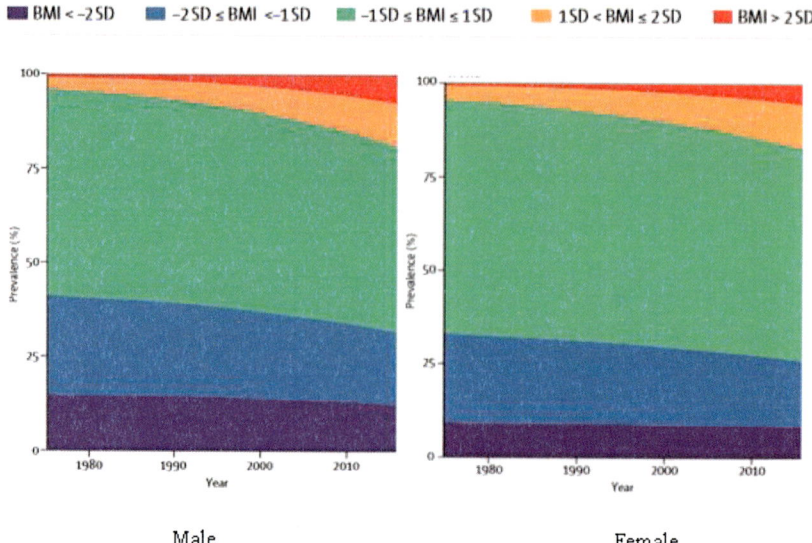

FIGURE 2-5 Trends in global age-standardized prevalence of body mass index (BMI) categories in male and female children and adolescents (aged 5–19 years).
SOURCES: NCD-RisC, 2017. Presented by Lindsay Jaacks, October 9, 2018. Reprinted with permission from Elsevier.

obesity, adding that disparities in prevalence occur both among and within countries.

Regarding geographic variation, Jaacks pointed to increases in the prevalence of overweight and obesity in both rural and urban areas of several major world regions. In approximately half of the countries analyzed, she elaborated, there were greater increases in rural than in urban areas (Jaacks et al., 2015). She focused on India as an example of a country that has a low national prevalence of obesity but substantial variation in within-state obesity prevalence. Appealing for more local data, she mentioned China, Nigeria, and the United States as other large countries with high subnational variability in obesity prevalence (CDC, 2017a; Kandala and Stranges, 2014; National Center for Chronic and Noncommunicable Disease Control and Prevention, 2016).

Jaacks went on to highlight recent estimates of the consequences of the global obesity epidemic. High BMI is among the top risk factors contributing to disability-adjusted life years in high-income countries, as well as across the world overall (GBD 2016 Risk Factor Collaborators, 2017), she reported. She cited as another consequence increasing loss of disease-free years as a person moves from normal to higher levels of BMI (Nyberg et al.,

2018). Third, she said, is a rise in diabetes mortality (IHME, 2018), and she cautioned that diabetes diagnoses will increase if the high-BMI epidemic is not controlled. "The health systems that we have been working with have no capacity to take on this high burden of diabetes," she warned.

Jaacks closed by reiterating the increasing burden of obesity in every region of the world, with data showing that 50 million girls, 74 million boys, 390 million women, and 281 million men were estimated to have obesity in 2016 (NCD-RisC, 2017).

OBESITY IN ASIAN POPULATIONS

Vasanti Malik, research scientist in the Department of Nutrition, Harvard T.H. Chan School of Public Health, discussed obesity trends in Asian populations. She opened by explaining that while obesity prevalence increased steadily across all global regions from 1975 to 2014, it remained lower in Asia than in other regions (see Figure 2-6). She reported that in India, according to Patel and colleagues (2015), obesity prevalence is higher in urban than in rural regions, but it is increasing in rural areas as well, particularly among adults. She cited other data indicating that the prevalence of overweight among Asians living in the United States is 27.5 percent, with variation among subgroups: it is highest among Asian Indian and Filipino populations and lower in East Asian populations, such as the Chinese (Barnes et al., 2008).

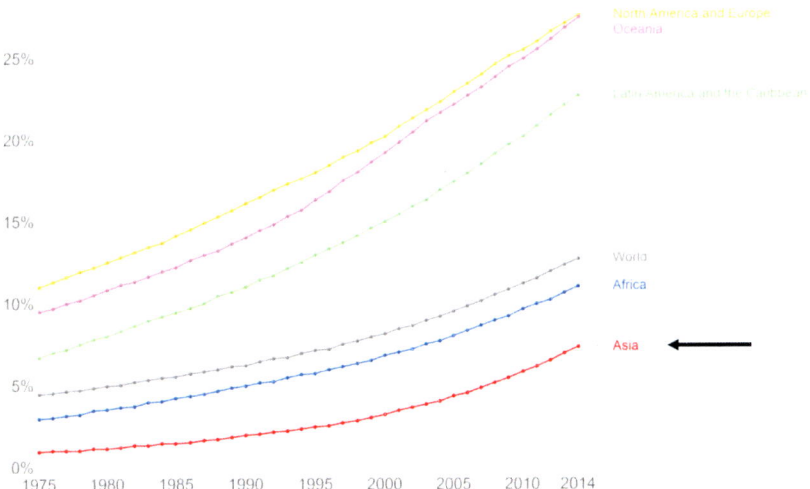

FIGURE 2-6 Prevalence of obesity (body mass index [BMI] >30) in adults (aged 18+ years) by world region.
SOURCES: Ritchie and Roser, 2018. Presented by Vasanti Malik, October 9, 2018.

Malik reminded participants that obesity is linked to a number of chronic diseases, elaborating in particular on its relationship with diabetes. Diabetes prevalence has increased across the globe, she noted, mirroring trends in obesity prevalence (see Figure 2-7). But she clarified that the relationship between obesity and diabetes is not consistent across populations, pointing to a comparison of the United States and eight Asian countries, among which India had the highest prevalence of type 2 diabetes but the lowest prevalence of obesity. This is not what one would expect to see, she observed, suggesting that it raises questions about the relationship between obesity and diabetes in Asian populations. She noted further that Asians develop diabetes at younger ages, illustrating this point with data showing that the prevalence of type 2 diabetes among 30- to 39-year-olds in Asian countries was higher than that among the same age group in the United States (Yoon et al., 2006).

The development of diabetes at younger ages may help explain its rapidly rising prevalence in Asian regions, Malik suggested. She displayed a map of worldwide adult diabetes prevalence for 2017, pointing out that prevalence is comparable in India and the United States (IDF, 2017). She also showed the projected increases in adult diabetes prevalence: the regions expected to experience the greatest rise between 2017 and 2045 are Southeast Asia (84 percent increase), the Middle East and North Africa (110 percent increase), and Africa (156 percent increase) (IDF, 2018). She characterized these projections as alarming, considering that many of these countries have the coexisting burden of undernutrition and health care systems that are not equipped to handle the increasing prevalence of diabetes.

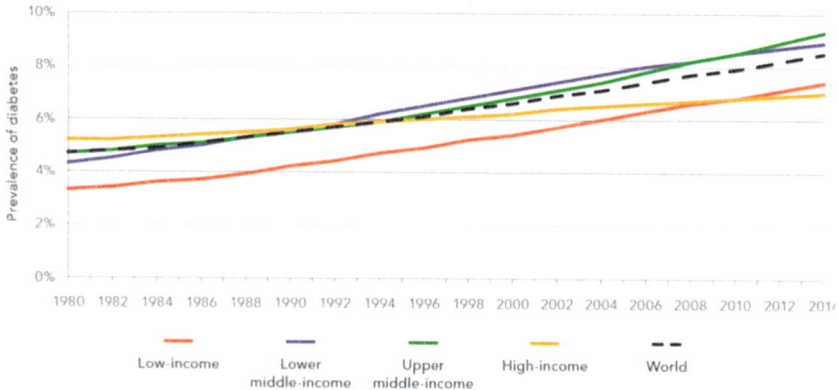

FIGURE 2-7 Global trends in type 2 diabetes prevalence.
SOURCES: WHO, 2016a. Presented by Vasanti Malik, October 9, 2018. Reprinted with permission from WHO.

Malik then highlighted the high prevalence of diabetes and cardiovascular risk factors in Asian populations, among whom the average BMI is below 25, the typical threshold for overweight. Yet, she added, while this is the threshold at which metabolic risk factors are observed among Western populations, the same is not necessarily the case among Asian populations. Some of these populations, especially South Asians, tend to have less muscle and more abdominal fat relative to white Europeans, she elaborated, so the same BMI may represent a higher percentage of body fat in the former than in the latter groups. According to Malik, these observations represent a limitation of BMI for assessing adiposity, but may help explain why diabetes tends to occur at lower BMIs and younger ages among Asian populations. She cited the example of two authors sharing the same BMI but differing in percentage of body fat.

Malik continued by reporting that WHO suggested lower BMI cutoff points for overweight and obesity in Asian populations (WHO Expert Consultation, 2004) because of their increased metabolic risk at lower BMIs (and younger ages) compared with Western populations. She pointed out that WHO's traditional overweight range is 25.0 to 29.9 kg/m^2, whereas for Asian populations, it is 23.0 to 27.4 kg/m^2; for obesity, the ranges are ≥30 kg/m^2 and for Asian populations, ≥27.5 kg/m^2. Ethnic-specific cutoff points have also been suggested for waist circumference (WHO, 2011), Malik added.

Malik explained that the concept of ethnic-specific BMI cutoff points has been informed by observations such as those of Deurenberg-Yap and colleagues (2000), who observed a paradox of low BMI and high body fat percentage among Asian subgroups living in Singapore. At the same BMI, she reported, Indians had the highest percentage of body fat, while Chinese had the lowest. These researchers suggested that for the same amount of body fat as Caucasians with a BMI of 30, the BMI cutoff points for obesity would be about 27 for Chinese and Malays and 26 for Indians.

Next, Malik showed data from Gujral and colleagues (2017), who examined the relationship among cardiometabolic abnormalities with normal-weight persons from five ethnic groups in the United States (white, Chinese American, African American, Hispanic, and South Asian). She reported that the prevalence of metabolic abnormalities within the normal-weight category was much higher in South Asians and Hispanics, followed by African Americans and Chinese Americans, compared with whites. The equivalent metabolic abnormalities observed among a white population with a BMI of 25, she elaborated, were observed at lower BMI cutoff points in the other ethnic groups, including as low as 19.6 for South Asians.

"This is telling us that BMI alone is not the best indicator of cardiometabolic risk in most of these Asian populations," she observed.

Similar findings have been observed in a different population, Malik continued, referencing a study of South Asian, Chinese, European, and

Aboriginal populations in Canada (Razak et al., 2007). For a given BMI, she said, elevated glucose and lipid factors were more likely to be present in South Asian, Chinese, and Aboriginal populations compared with Europeans. According to these researchers, she added, the cutoff point for defining obesity is lower by approximately 6 kg/m² among non-European groups.

Malik went on to discuss a recent prospective cohort study in India in which significant ethnic differences in the prevalence of type 2 diabetes without excess weight were observed (Gujral et al., 2018). Compared with a white American population, the Asian population experienced higher diabetes prevalence at underweight and normal weight, she elaborated, commenting that diabetes is not seen among the underweight population of white men, and its prevalence is very low in underweight white women. She added that an increased risk for diabetes has also been observed at lower levels of BMI in migrant South Asian groups compared with white individuals or Europeans (Sattar and Gill, 2015). In summary, she said, South Asians develop diabetes at lower weights, at younger ages, and more rapidly (with regard to the progression from impaired glucose tolerance to diabetes) compared with their white counterparts. She stressed the implications of these findings for prevention strategies in Asia, as well as among migrant populations living in the United States and other countries.

Data on the relationship between BMI and metabolic risk among children are sparse, Malik continued. She cited one study that examined differences in body composition and metabolic status between white children in the United Kingdom and Asian Indian children in India. She reported that, despite having lower BMIs, the Indian children had greater adiposity than the white children, and they were also more insulin resistant even after adjustment for adiposity (Lakshmi et al., 2012). However, given the paucity of data, Malik suggested that more research in this area may be useful.

Malik ended by noting that diabetes costs many countries more than $10 billion annually (IDF, 2018), underscoring the importance of obesity and diabetes prevention strategies. Asia's coexisting problem with underweight has implications for obesity policy, she added. Finally, she proposed incorporating Asian-specific BMI and waist circumference cutoff points in screening programs to help reduce the diabetes burden in Asian populations around the globe.

OBESITY IN AFRICAN MIGRANT AND NONMIGRANT POPULATIONS

The world is experiencing rapid ethnic diversification due to an increase in international migration, said Karlijn Meeks, postdoctoral research fellow in the Department of Public Health, Academic Medical Center, University of Amsterdam. According to the United Nations (2017a), she reported, there were about 173 million international migrants in 2000 and 258 million in 2017. High-income countries host about two-thirds of all migrants, she added, and one in three people is of migrant descent in large European cities such as Amsterdam and London.

Meeks outlined three methods for assessing migrant health. The first and most commonly used is to compare the migrant population with the host population, looking at ethnic differences or ethnic inequalities. The second method is to compare the same migrant group living in different countries, studying the role of national context. And the third is to compare members of a migrant group with their compatriots who have not migrated, studying the role of migration.

As an example of the first method, Meeks pointed to HELIUS (Healthy Life in an Urban Setting), a large cohort study that compared five ethnic minority groups in Amsterdam with the Dutch host population. She reported that all five ethnic minority groups were more affected by overweight and obesity compared with the Dutch, with the highest rates of overweight and obesity being seen in the populations of African descent (Snijder et al., 2017).

Migrants' destinations matter, Meeks stressed, because the prevalence of overweight and obesity varies widely among high-income countries based on Organisation for Economic Co-operation and Development (OECD, 2017) health statistics. The national context differs in these countries in ways that can influence socioeconomic status, lifestyle, the food environment, and access to health care, she elaborated. Thus, she suggested, comparing the same migrant group across different countries can help pinpoint the contextual factors that drive increased risk for overweight and obesity, findings that can benefit both the migrant and host populations.

To illustrate the second method, which entails exploring how national context influences health behaviors, Meeks displayed data from the Netherlands and England on the prevalence of tobacco smoking. The prevalence of smoking is higher in the Netherlands among the Dutch than in England among the English, she pointed out, and the same pattern is reflected in the migrant populations living in these countries: a higher prevalence of smoking among African migrants living in the Netherlands compared with African migrants living in England, and a higher prevalence among Indian migrants living in the Netherlands compared with Indian migrants living in England (Agyemang et al., 2010).

Meeks then turned to the third method, which involves studying the role of migration, which she said is important for both migrant populations and nonmigrants. Comparing migrant populations with their compatriots who have not migrated, she explained, can reveal lifestyle changes that occurred upon migration, and help identify key predisposing factors for increased risk of overweight and obesity. She pointed out that migrant populations take results of studies comparing them with their nonmigrant compatriots more seriously than those comparing them with host populations, which they may perceive as unfair. Results are also important to nonmigrant populations, she added, because rapid changes in lifestyle and urbanization experienced by migrants in host countries likely reflect what is happening in low- and middle-income countries and can help forecast future health threats to the nonmigrants.

To illustrate the role of migration, Meeks shared data on the prevalence of overweight and obesity for two different age groups of adult male and female Ghanaians living in three locations. In each age and sex group, prevalence was lowest in rural Ghana, higher in urban Ghana, and highest in the Netherlands, reaching 95 percent among Ghanaian women over age 40 living in Amsterdam (see Figure 2-8).

Meeks next presented insights from the Research on Obesity and Diabetes among African Migrants (RODAM) study, which examined the roles of both migration and national context (Agyemang et al., 2016). Data were collected for nearly 6,400 Ghanaians in 5 locations: residents of rural and urban Ghana and migrants living in London, Berlin, and Amsterdam. Meeks reported that, for both men and women, the prevalence of overweight and obesity (BMI ≥25), obesity only (BMI ≥30), and abdominal obesity (waist circumference >102 cm in men and >88 cm in women) was lowest in rural Ghana, higher in urban Ghana, and highest in the three European cities. According to Meeks, migration played a larger role than national context; however, context played a role as well, given that there was about a 10 percent higher prevalence of overweight and obesity among Ghanaians (both men and women) living in London than in Berlin, for example (see Figure 2-9).

Meeks also pointed to the lower burden of overweight and obesity among Ghanaians in Ghana, based on data published in 2009 (see Figure 2-8), noting that the prevalence of obesity and overweight in urban Ghanaian women was closer to the prevalence in Europe (see Figure 2-9). While the prevalence of overweight, obesity, and abdominal obesity was higher among women than among men in all five locations, she reported, the prevalence of type 2 diabetes was higher among men in every location except rural Ghana (see Figure 2-10).

Meeks echoed Malik's observation regarding the existence of ethnic differences in the relationship between obesity and health outcomes such as diabetes. She showed data illustrating the positive relationship between BMI and the probability of diabetes among men in the five locations. Among men with the same BMI, the probability of developing diabetes varied by location, she observed, highlighting an example in which the probability was higher in Berlin than in rural Ghana. There was also a positive relationship between waist circumference and the probability of developing

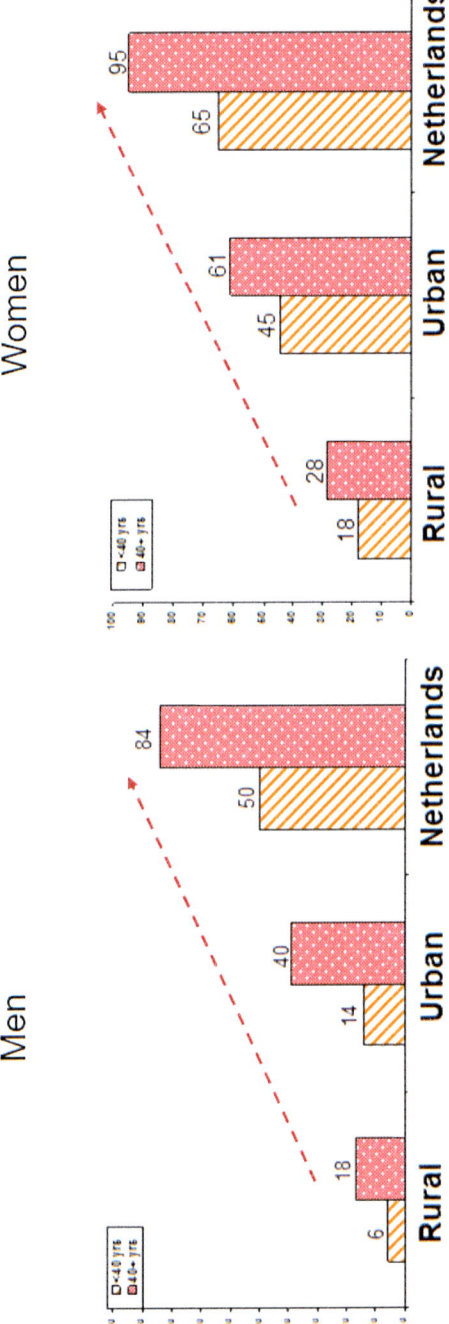

FIGURE 2-8 Ghanaians' prevalence of overweight and obesity (body mass index [BMI] ≥25) by age and location.
SOURCES: Agyemang et al., 2009. Presented by Karlijn Meeks, October 9, 2018. Reprinted with permission from Cambridge University Press.

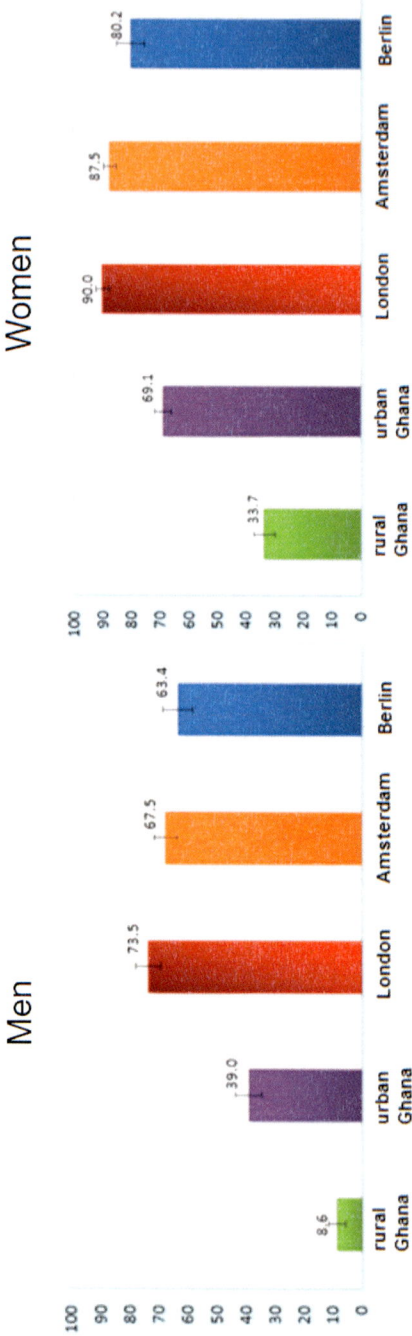

FIGURE 2-9 Ghanaians' age-standardized prevalence of overweight and obesity (body mass index [BMI] ≥25) by locality.
SOURCES: Agyemang et al., 2016. Presented by Karlijn Meeks, October 9, 2018. Reprinted with permission from BioMed Central.

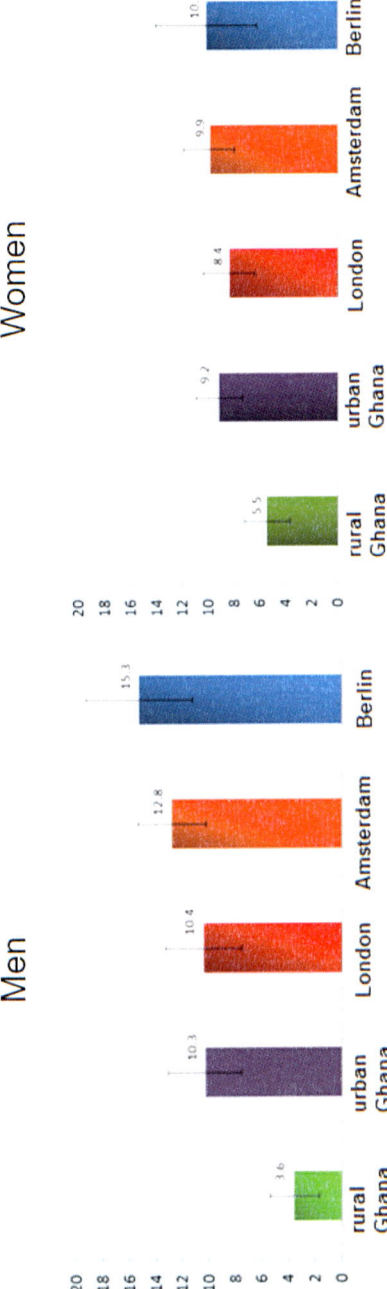

FIGURE 2-10 Ghanaians' age-standardized prevalence of type 2 diabetes (World Health Organization criteria) by locality.
SOURCES: Agyemang et al., 2016. Presented by Karlijn Meeks, October 9, 2018. Reprinted with permission from BioMed Central.

diabetes, she stated, with similar patterns for women. "This clearly illustrates the role of national context beyond just BMI," she maintained.

To unravel the contributors to overweight and obesity in the RODAM study population, Meeks briefly discussed environmental, genetic, and epigenetic factors. Environmental factors, such as the food environment and diet, physical activity, and stress, she said, differ by national context and can increase the risk of overweight and obesity in migrants compared with nonmigrants. Turning to genetics, she explained that more than 80 loci have been associated with polygenic obesity, but these loci explain only a small fraction of heritability (Locke et al., 2015). More important, she added, data on African populations are limited: only 19 percent of genetic studies are performed in non-European populations, and a majority of that segment consists of Asian populations (Popejoy and Fullerton, 2016). Finally, she observed that lifestyle can affect epigenetics, the cellular mechanisms that regulate gene expression. She cited as an example that if a person starts smoking or makes dietary or physical activity changes, that behavior can induce epigenetic changes that may increase health risk. According to Meeks, while the RODAM study described novel loci associated with obesity in its Ghanaian cohort (Meeks et al., 2017), more research could help determine whether certain environmental factors drive these epigenetic changes to increase the risk of overweight and obesity, or if overweight and obesity induce the epigenetic changes and thereby increase the risk for other diseases.

In summary, Meeks pointed to the high burden of overweight and obesity among African migrants in Europe and an increasing burden in the African region. She added that obesity is an independent risk factor for diabetes, but context matters, and she highlighted the importance of unraveling the complex interplay between genetic and environmental factors as determinants of obesity in Africans.

THE DOUBLE BURDEN OF MALNUTRITION

According to Rachel Nugent, vice president for noncommunicable diseases (NCDs), RTI International, it is important to include the double burden of malnutrition in the conversation about global obesity. Also known as the "dual burden," the concept of the double burden is relatively new and underresearched, she observed, so a number of its important aspects are not fully described.

Nugent explained that the double burden refers to the simultaneous presence of undernutrition (one or more of stunting, wasting, and micronutrient deficiencies) and overweight/obesity, and can be measured at the individual, household, regional, and national levels. According to the Food and Agriculture Organization of the United Nations (FAO), undernutrition affects an estimated 800 million people worldwide, while the problem of overweight and obesity affects 2 billion people (FAO et al., 2018; WHO, 2018b). In 2014, the Second International Congress on Nutrition framed the issue as malnutrition in all its forms, Nugent said, and she suggested that this broad vision of malnutrition is helping to motivate research on the topic. FAO and WHO are also perpetuating this framing, she noted, and it is gaining greater acceptance, although many of the relationships between undernutrition and overweight and obesity are not yet fully understood.

Nugent shared unpublished maps showing where the double burden of malnutrition is found. She explained that its extent varies depending on the selection of criteria for undernutrition and prevalence of overweight and obesity. At the countrywide level, only a few countries experience a high (40 percent) prevalence of overweight and obesity alongside high levels of undernutrition, she said. But she explained that the two conditions coexist in more countries when the definition is based on a lower prevalence (20 or 30 percent) of overweight and obesity and a broader definition of undernutrition. According to Nugent, this variability reflects the lack of a firm definition for the problem. She added that if subnational-level data were being considered instead of only national-level data, the double burden of malnutrition would appear in even more places.

Nugent went on to explore the drivers and conditions associated with the double burden. She referred to a figure originally developed to examine the drivers of cardiovascular disease (see Figure 2-11), which she said conveys that many environmental drivers are related to diet and to factors upstream from food systems and agriculture. If one examines the changes over time in dietary behaviors and intake patterns, she observed, warning signs emerge along the way. She also argued that shifts in the global food system, such as the commercial sector's increasing influence over the nutrition conditions in many countries, contribute to the environmental factors that are associated with increases in overweight and obesity alongside continued undernutrition. In addition, she said, it is challenging to measure consumption of processed food accurately. Based on available data, she highlighted a trend of increasing volumes of retail and food service sales for sugar-sweetened beverages and "junk foods" in Chile, Malaysia, and South Africa (Euromonitor, 2018).

Nugent then transitioned to the economic costs of the double burden, first acknowledging that the economic literature on the topic is sparse. This is because the heterogeneity across economic studies of underweight and of overweight and obesity makes it challenging to combine the literature, she explained. She added that only two studies have examined the economic costs of both undernutrition and overweight and obesity, and emphasized that common measures for the two conditions do not exist. For example, she elaborated, the impact of undernutrition may be based on the risk of disease attributable to undernutrition or on educational attainment related

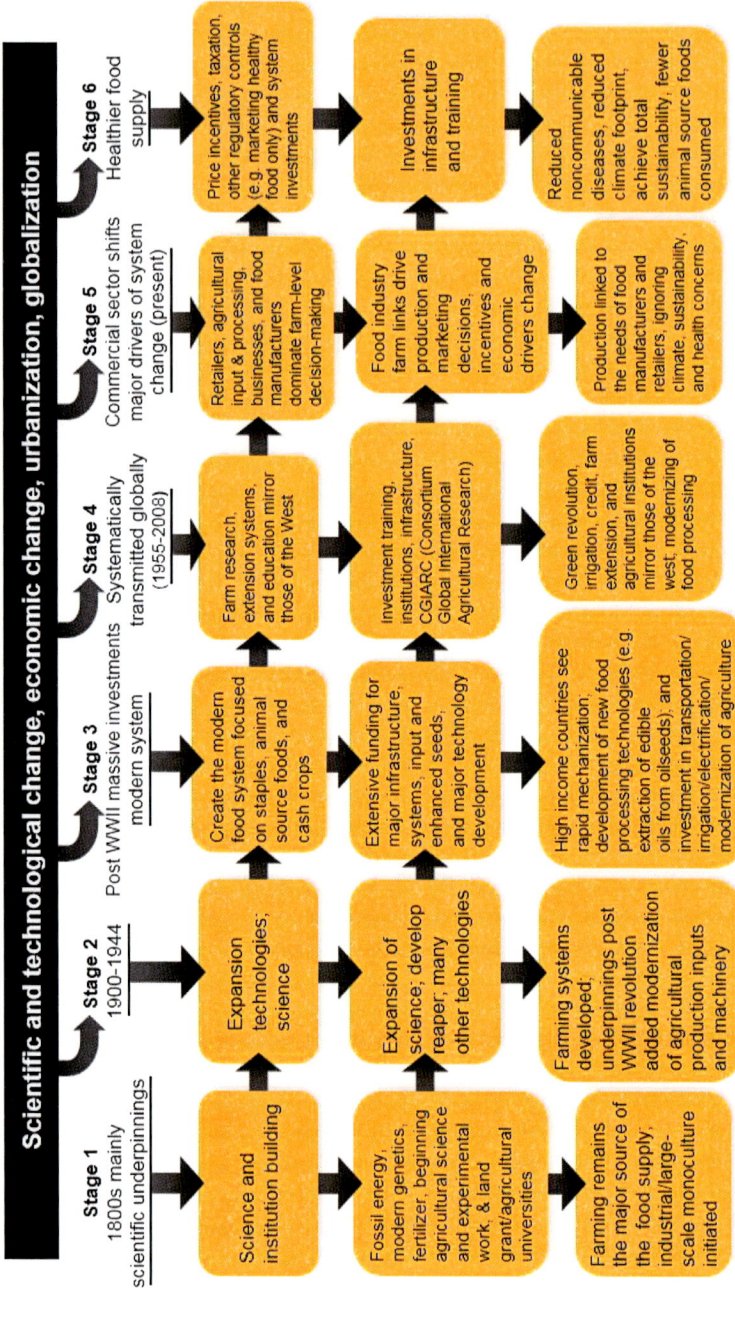

FIGURE 2-11 Drivers and conditions associated with the double burden: stages of modern agricultural and food system development.
SOURCES: Anand et al., 2015. Presented by Rachel Nugent, October 9, 2018.

to undernutrition, while the cost of obesity is typically measured in medical expenditures and productivity losses.

In one of the above two studies, Nugent reported, the Economic Commission for Latin America and the Caribbean (ECLAC, 2016) considered multiple pathways to measure the projected costs of undernutrition and overweight and obesity over 65 years in three countries. The study found a total cost ranging from 0.2 percent of GDP in Chile (all from obesity) to 4.3 percent of GDP in Ecuador (2.6 percent from undernutrition and 1.7 percent from obesity). Nugent observed that the study's method of measuring and combining two different phenomena was "a far from perfect way of measuring the double burden of malnutrition, but it's the best that could be done."

In the second study, Nugent continued, conducted in China and India, it was estimated that in 1993, the cost of NCDs due to under- and overnutrition amounted to about 1.1 percent and 2.1 percent of GDP in India and China, respectively (Popkin et al., 2001). When the estimate for China was updated, she noted, the cost was 4 percent of GDP in 2000 and projected to reach 9 percent by 2025 (Popkin et al., 2006). Despite the lack of both modeling capacity and empirical data, she argued "we can feel pretty certain that there is a significant economic impact from both of these conditions."

Nugent then cited a number of "double-duty" interventions that can address all forms of malnutrition, adding the caveat that while there is evidence for their impact on one or another form of malnutrition, evidence demonstrating their impact on the double burden is lacking (Shekar et al., 2017; WCRFI, 2018; WHO, 2017). She highlighted three interventions that were chosen for economic analysis based on the ability to get strong data (i.e., data for which there is confidence in the effect sizes, although effects are not necessarily large) for their impact on both undernutrition and overweight/obesity: breastfeeding promotion, school nutrition programs, and food advertising.

To close, Nugent recapped some of the challenges associated with the double burden: a complex set of drivers and conditions, uneven and noncomparable data sources on forms of malnutrition (with much more information available on undernutrition than on overweight and obesity, particularly in developing countries), intergenerational factors that are both epigenetic and environmental, and different outcome measures that reflect the various impacts of malnutrition across the life cycle. Most important, she asserted, is the lack of evidence from double-duty interventions and programs (Ruel and Alderman, 2013).

DISCUSSION

During a discussion period following the four presentations summarized above, speakers discussed how to better design programs and policy interventions and addressed questions from the audience on epigenetics and environments, food systems, cultural food practices, and trade issues.

Program and Policy Interventions

The four speakers shared ideas for improving the design of programs and policy strategies to address overweight and obesity. Nugent suggested designing interventions that address malnutrition in all its forms. From the perspective of the double burden, she explained, "there is some evidence that we have been causing harm in different parts of the world, where our historical knowledge base and our paradigms are to address undernutrition." She cited that as a result of the nutrition community's focus on the various forms of undernutrition, it has been late in realizing the harms caused by changes in environments and food systems. "So we're really behind the eight ball on addressing the obesity and overweight problem," she said. She cautioned that basing actions on national data could exacerbate the problem in places where a coexisting burden of underweight and overweight/obesity is apparent only after one looks at subnational data. She urged stakeholders to make programming, funding, and policy decisions that consider malnutrition in all its forms.

Jaacks concurred with Nugent, adding that "the focus has been on undernourishment for so long, and undernourishment continues to be a problem, so you can't divert all resources to overweight and obesity." She agreed that collecting more local-level data is critical to identify the problem in a given location—whether undernutrition, overweight and obesity, or both—so that programs and policies can be designed accordingly. Economos advocated for more frequent data collection, adding that "we can't look at data from 10 years ago and design programs."

To address migrant health, Meeks proposed moving beyond the common assessment method of comparing migrants with their host population. She acknowledged that "many of those studies show indeed a higher burden in the migrant population," but, she argued, "to really pinpoint what underlying factors are driving this increased risk, we need to look at other designs as well," such as those that examine the roles of national context and migration. Genetic, epigenetic, and other underlying factors could explain different rates of certain health outcomes in migrants, she added. Economos suggested that qualitative data could provide additional information about what is going on in a specific population and context.

Malik suggested that an important step toward prevention would be for screening programs to adopt lower BMI cutoff points for Asian populations in the United States and in other high-income countries. She reminded participants that diabetes and other metabolic risk factors develop at lower BMI levels in Asian populations, and thus early intervention is important. She also called for more research to better understand the relationship between body fat and BMI in children. Jaacks mentioned that the American Diabetes Association has adopted a lower BMI cutoff point at which Asian Americans are screened for diabetes.

Epigenetics and Environments

In response to a participant's question about whether epigenetic changes varied across the RODAM study cohort in the three European countries, Meeks replied that the small sample size of the study cohort that included epigenetic data precluded an examination of epigenetic differences among the European contexts. She noted, however, that her group has compared the epigenetic profiles of Ghanaians in rural Ghana, urban Ghana, and Europe and found that across the genome, many loci differed among those locations. The different environmental factors in those sites is "triggering immense epigenetic changes," she asserted, and suggested that environmental factors are likely increasing Ghanaians' disease risk in the European settings.

Food Systems

A participant asked for examples of farming and food distribution practices that countries are implementing to address the double burden. Nugent replied that a field of study called "nutrition-sensitive agriculture" seeks to identify methods for changing agriculture and food systems; she also noted that agriculture programs and studies are not designed to measure nutrition and health outcomes. Notwithstanding the lack of strong evidence of causal connections, she continued, there is reasonably good evidence that improving the processes along the value chain of food production and distribution can deliver healthier food to people. Regarding "upstream" approaches to improve the food system, she suggested considering subsidy, tax, and trade policies that provide incentives to farmers and others in the food system and ultimately support healthier food production and distribution practices. She urged a more "cohesive, integrative way of thinking about these things, because it's all connected." Economos underscored the complexity and nonlinearity of food system processes, and Jaacks added that the conversations around agriculture policy are even more complicated in low- and middle-income countries. In India, she observed, the vast majority of farmers own less than 1 hectare of land, so the large-scale, national policies that are discussed for higher-income countries are not as applicable.

Another participant asked Malik to shed light on the continued use of BMI as a screening indicator, particularly for diabetes, and wondered whether a transition to body fat percentage had been considered. Malik replied that the use of waist circumference (as a measure of abdominal adiposity) has been discussed, but a challenge is that it is more complicated to measure, while measurement of BMI is relatively straightforward. Nonetheless, she believes that "waist circumference, if measured properly, would be a better indicator of adiposity." Jaacks agreed that measuring waist circumference in the field is difficult, and stated that the tools currently available for the purpose would make it difficult to collect such data at the population level.

Cultural Food Practices

According to Meeks, migrants may retain food practices from their home countries even if those practices are no longer suited to their new context. As an example, she recounted a national campaign advocating palm oil consumption in Ghana to help remediate the country's high rate of vitamin A deficiency. Ghanaian migrants in Europe remembered that campaign, she said, and continued to use palm oil, which is high in saturated fat, even though vitamin A deficiency is uncommon in that region. Malik suggested that additional qualitative research could help clarify the factors influencing dietary choices and inform interventions to improve diet quality. Nugent asserted that qualitative research could help in understanding a culture's food behaviors and values-driven attachment to certain traditional foods, even though food consumption data may suggest that these foods are no longer commonly consumed.

Trade Issues

A participant claimed that rates of chronic disease were lower in some populations when mostly traditional foods were consumed, and asked whether there have been global efforts to help lower-income countries prevent the importation of highly processed foods. Nugent replied that overall, trade has generally had a positive effect on nutrition, although she acknowledged the complexity of the relationships among trade issues, food consumption, and health outcomes.

3

Global Obesity Prevention and Treatment Efforts

Highlights from the Presentations of Individual Speakers

- The purpose of the World Obesity Federation's Management Advocacy for Providers, Patients, and Systems program is to gather intelligence on in-country health care systems and practices for obesity policy, prevention, and treatment. The most frequently reported barrier to obesity treatment is a lack of training for health care providers. (Olivia Barata Cavalcanti)
- More than one-quarter of adults globally do not achieve recommended levels of physical activity. The World Health Organization produced a global action plan on physical activity for 2018–2030 to accelerate the implementation of policies to create active societies, active environments, active people, and active systems. (Fiona Bull)
- Eating ultraprocessed products is associated with poorer dietary quality and promotion of obesity. Regulation of the advertising and marketing of these products, as is seen in some Latin American and Caribbean countries, is suggested to help solve the obesity problem. (Fabio da Silva Gomes)

The charge to the three speakers in the workshop's second session was to highlight efforts to identify, promote, and monitor global policy and systems initiatives that are designed to address the obesity problem, said session moderator James Sallis, distinguished professor emeritus of family medicine and public health at the University of California, San Diego, and professorial fellow at Australian Catholic University, Melbourne.

MANAGEMENT AND ADVOCACY FOR PROVIDERS, PATIENTS, AND SYSTEMS

Olivia Barata Cavalcanti, director of health systems and professional education at the World Obesity Federation, discussed her organization's Management Advocacy for Providers, Patients, and Systems (MAPPS) program. She described the program's main goal as learning how national health care systems function regarding obesity policy, prevention, and treatment. The findings will be used to create a Health Systems for Obesity Index, she said, which will be added to the Federation's Global Obesity Observatory, a repository of obesity prevalence and incidence data.

Barata Cavalcanti explained that the World Obesity Federation decided to focus on health systems because obesity is being tackled with multi-factorial solutions. It is helpful to understand the clinical environment in different countries, she added, and whether and how individuals can access obesity treatment. She argued that identifying barriers and potential solutions to overcome them can lead to best practices that can be shared with other countries.

Barata Cavalcanti shared a brief description of the MAPPS methodology. The program began by convening a group of health systems experts to advise the process. Data collection commenced with an online literature review in PubMed, using selected search keywords in combination with the country's name to learn more about its health systems in relation to obesity treatment and control strategies. The team implemented narrower search terms when results were too numerous, and used more location-specific terms as the search progressed. A website scoping review followed, Barata Cavalcanti continued, whereby the team explored, for example, the websites of ministries of health for different countries. The team also performed keyword searches to find information about health systems' financial mechanisms for coverage of obesity treatment. According to Barata Cavalcanti, limitations included language barriers that made it difficult to extract materials not in English, as well as an overabundance of materials in English, which required limiting the depth of the research. She added that the quality and quantity of information varied among countries, and the team frequently had to conduct interviews with in-country informants to validate findings. These interviews contributed additional value, she remarked, because they provided on-the-ground perspectives on how the various health systems work.

Next, Barata Cavalcanti continued, the team sent questionnaires to key informants in each country of interest. The aim, she explained, was to collect information about such topics as whether the country defines obesity as a disease, the operations and funding mechanisms for its health care system, and cultural and political influences on obesity. "We had some difficulty getting responses," she disclosed, suggesting that this was likely because the questionnaire was lengthy. Furthermore, recipients included people in high-level positions, she observed, "which means that they are also very busy."

The team then decided to develop two shorter, online questionnaires, Barata Cavalcanti reported, giving recipients the choice of participating in an in-depth interview. Since then, she said, in addition to the World Obesity Federation's country members, more than 100 key informants have been invited to complete the online questionnaires. She added that respondents include a variety of medical and health care professionals, public health advisors, and researchers, to provide a "360-degree perspective." The questionnaires have been translated into Italian, Portuguese, and Spanish, which she said is expected to improve the response rate.

Barata Cavalcanti shared the preliminary results of this work, remarking that they are constantly updated and refined as more countries and stakeholders are added. To gauge progress toward defining obesity as a disease, she explained, interviewees are asked to rate on a scale from 0 to 10 where their country's government and health care providers are in that process. Every country is at a different place in this journey, she noted, and results are not consistent among high-income or low-income countries. What is consistent, she reported, is that health care providers are more likely than government officials to rate their country as being further along in the process. Some interviewees from the same country had completely different perspectives depending on their line of work and location within the country, she added, and outliers were removed from the results.

Barata Cavalcanti highlighted as one of the most valuable results of the study that interviewees identified their country's five greatest barriers to obesity treatment. Lack of training for health care providers was the most commonly cited barrier, which was named by 50 percent of respondents, followed by lack of access to treatment and medications (especially subsidized medication) and lack of knowledge and awareness (among the public, health care providers, the government, and patients) about obesity's causes and impact. Additional barriers identified are shown in Figure 3-1.

Barata Cavalcanti also shared data on the availability of specialized obesity training in 30 countries: approximately one-quarter of the countries have no such specialist training available; in another quarter, the availability of such training is unknown; and the remaining half of the countries reported specialist training for bariatric surgery, nutrition, counseling, or other broad-ranging specialist training. Barata Cavalcanti observed that the diversity of responses indicates the lack of a consistent plan of action for tackling obesity among different health systems. "That is one of the biggest problems that we have at the moment," she maintained. She added that

Biggest barriers to obesity treatment

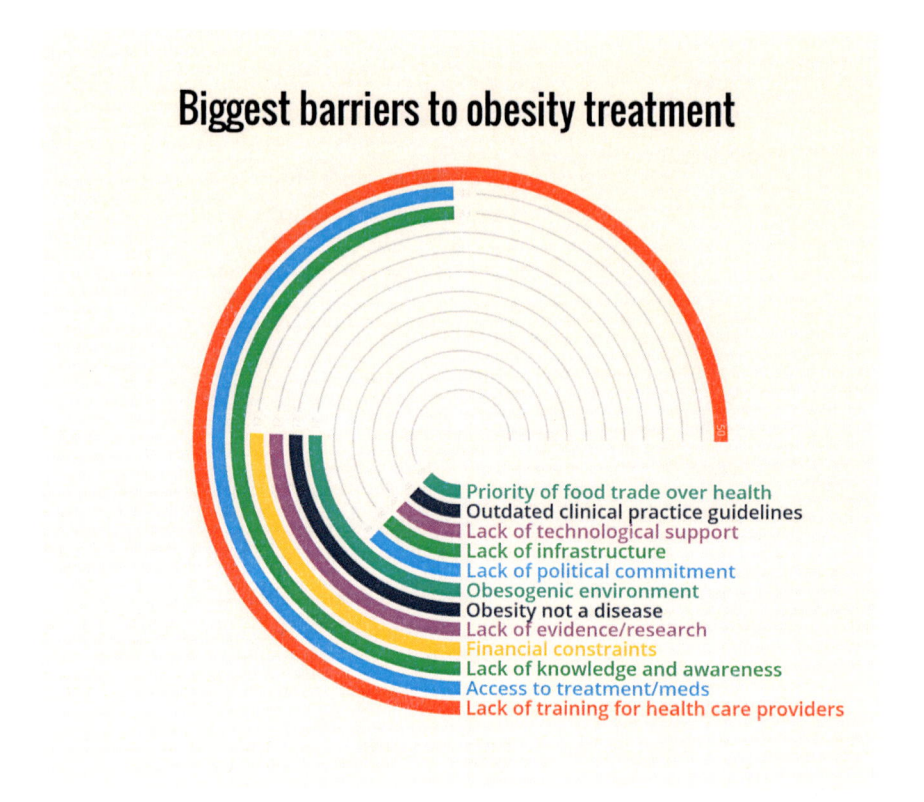

- Priority of food trade over health
- Outdated clinical practice guidelines
- Lack of technological support
- Lack of infrastructure
- Lack of political commitment
- Obesogenic environment
- Obesity not a disease
- Lack of evidence/research
- Financial constraints
- Lack of knowledge and awareness
- Access to treatment/meds
- Lack of training for health care providers

FIGURE 3-1 Greatest barriers to obesity treatment, as reported by the World Obesity Federation.
NOTE: Numbers at the end of each arc represent the percentage of respondents identifying that factor as a barrier.
SOURCE: Presented by Olivia Barata Cavalcanti, October 9, 2018.

lower availability of qualified obesity treatment professionals was reported in rural compared with urban areas.

Results of the data analyses are shared with country governments in the form of "traffic light report cards," Barata Cavalcanti said (see Figure 3-2). The colors indicate areas in which a country is doing well and those in which it can improve, she explained, adding that there is wide variability among countries.

MORE ACTIVE PEOPLE FOR A HEALTHIER WORLD

Fiona Bull, program manager in the Department of Prevention of Noncommunicable Diseases at the World Health Organization (WHO),

Where is your country's government in the journey toward defining "Obesity as a disease"? (🟢: Defined as disease, 🟡: Partial, 🔴: No, ⚪: Not known)	🔴
Where is your country's health care provider in the journey toward defining "Obesity as a disease"? (🟢: Defined as disease, 🟡: Partial, 🔴: No, ⚪: Not known)	🔴
Do obesity treatment financing mechanisms facilitate equitable access to care? (e.g., is obesity treatment largely covered by out of pocket expense, insurance, or government health provision?) (🟢: Government, 🟡: Insurance, 🔴: Out of pocket expense, ⚪: Not known)	🔴
At what level of obesity are people usually eligible to access health care? (🟢: BMI ≥30, 🟡: ≥ 35, 🔴: ≥35 + co-morbidities or ≥ 40 kg/m^2, ⚪: not defined or not known)	⚪
Is there a system for training health professionals in recognizing obesity, its prevention, and its management? (🟢: Yes, 🟡: Partial, 🔴: No, ⚪: Not known)	🔴

FIGURE 3-2 Example of a country report card in the World Obesity Federation's Management Advocacy for Providers, Patients, and Systems (MAPPS) program.
NOTE: BMI = body mass index.
SOURCE: Presented by Olivia Barata Cavalcanti, October 9, 2018.

described the role of physical activity in obesity solutions and reviewed WHO's global action plan for increasing physical activity (WHO, 2018a).

Bull began with a brief review of key milestones in physical activity, noncommunicable diseases (NCDs), and global health, noting that "it has been a patchy history." A U.S. Surgeon General's report in 1996 "really put the stamp on physical activity," she asserted (HHS, 1996). The WHO Global Strategy on Diet, Physical Activity, and Health followed in 2004 (WHO, 2004), along with documents to help countries implement its guidance. As researchers and entities such as WHO made the case for physical activity's contributions to promoting health and preventing NCDs and obesity, things started to change, Bull recalled.

According to Bull, physical activity gained a "good foothold" with the 2013 release of WHO's *Global Action Plan for the Prevention and Control of NCDs 2013–2020* (WHO, 2013). That document, she elaborated, includes recommendations for policy actions to promote physical activity and sets a global target for a 10 percent relative reduction in the prevalence of insufficient physical activity by 2025. One of the report's appendixes presents "best buys" and "good buys," which she described as cost-effective interventions relevant for all countries, as determined by WHO-CHOICE (CHOosing Interventions that are Cost-Effective) cost-effective analysis methods, and which were updated in 2018. Bull explained that a "best buy" is public education campaigns combined with community-based education and environmental programs, and a "good buy" is counseling and referral as part of routine primary health care services through the use of brief interventions. Other interventions have not undergone the WHO-CHOICE cost-effectiveness modeling but are recognized as necessary and valuable, she pointed out, citing the examples of efforts to promote physical activity in school settings and to improve urban designs so as to provide safe, easy access to public transport. Most recently and after much consultation, she said, WHO produced a *Global Action Plan on Physical Activity 2018–2030* to accelerate implementation of the recommended policies (WHO, 2018a).

Bull paused to share the latest physical activity data released from WHO (Guthold et al., 2018), noting that these data "emphasize how countries were quite right in the urgent need to act." She stressed that 28 percent of adults globally fail to achieve the levels of physical activity recommended for optimal health. This percentage has been relatively unchanged since 2001, she observed, and the trend has remained flat for both men and women, with approximately 25 percent and 31 percent, respectively, not meeting recommended levels. Turning to regional differences in the current prevalence of inactivity, she flagged the Latin American and Caribbean region for its overall high levels of inactivity and sizable difference between men and women (see Figure 3-3). There is even more concern within regions, she added, noting that as many as 70 percent of people in some regions do not meet the recommendations.

Bull also pointed out that the prevalence of inactivity is lowest in low-income countries, higher in middle-income countries, and highest in high-income countries (see Figure 3-4). The pattern, she elaborated, shows that sedentary time is positively associated with urbanization and globalization and the corresponding changes to work and travel patterns. "We see this very profoundly in these data," she said.

Turning back to WHO's global action plan on physical activity, Bull highlighted the extensive multisector stakeholder consultation that was part of its development. She stated that this collaboration to determine what is feasible, practical, and applicable is expected to pay off in the implementation phase. Now that the plan has reached the milestone of World Health Assembly endorsement, she remarked that "in some ways, it is the end of the beginning."

Bull underscored the plan's message that there are many ways to be active. She added that talking about specific ways, such as playing, dancing, cycling, or walking, resonates with nonhealth sectors that may be less accustomed to the term "physical activity." She explained that the updated plan maintains the 2013 plan's global target of a 10 percent relative reduction in the prevalence of insufficient physical activity by 2025, and also targets a 15 percent reduction by 2030. To achieve these goals, she suggested that all people have access to safe and enabling environments, as well as

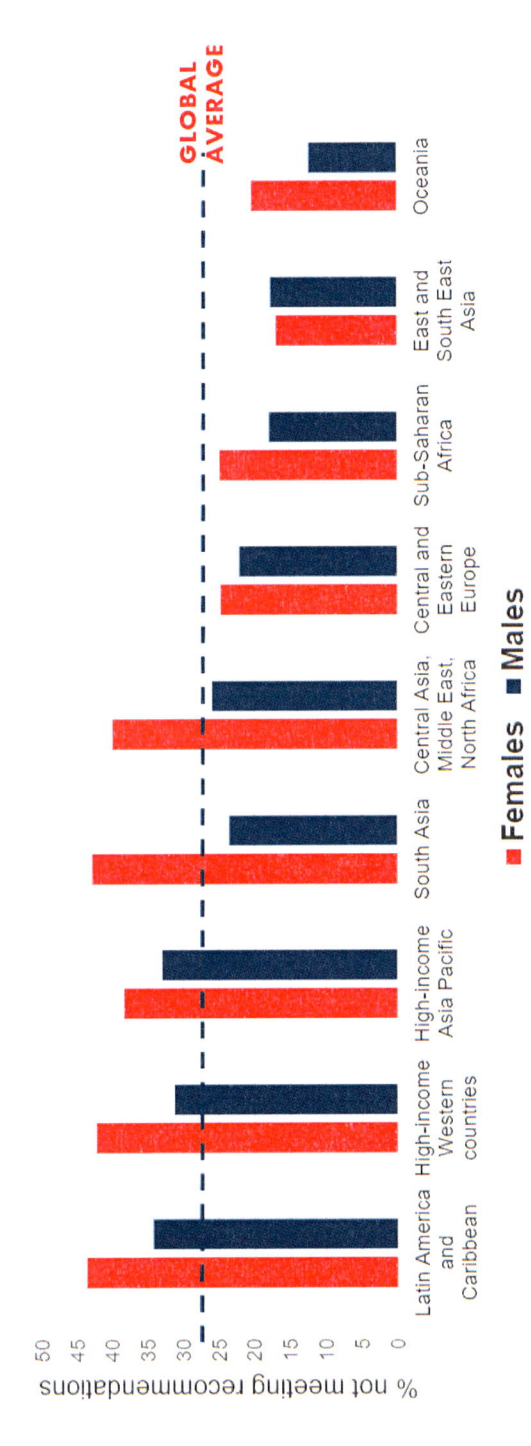

FIGURE 3-3 Percentage of people who do not meet physical activity recommendations, by sex and global region.
SOURCES: Adapted from Guthold et al., 2018. Presented by Fiona Bull on October 9, 2018. Reprinted with permission from Elsevier.

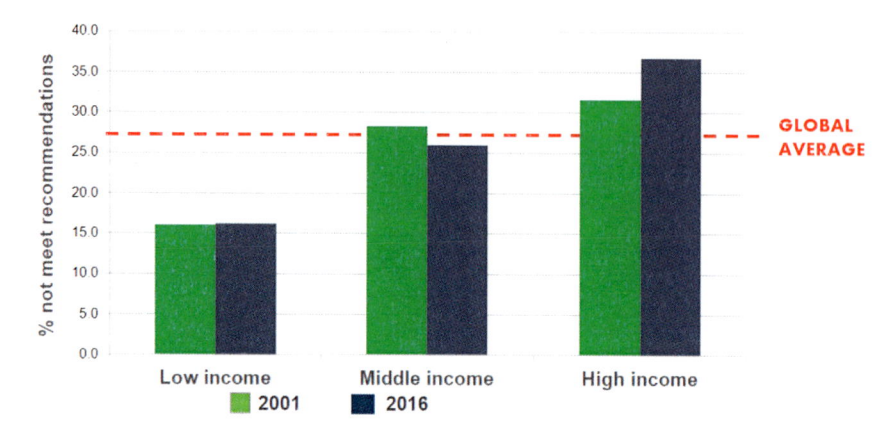

FIGURE 3-4 Percentage of people who do not meet physical activity recommendations, by World Bank income classification.
SOURCES: Adapted from Guthold et al., 2018. Presented by Fiona Bull on October 9, 2018. Reprinted with permission from Elsevier.

diverse opportunities to be physically active in their daily lives. She insisted that "one without the other will not be effective."

Bull then outlined the plan's four strategic objectives, each supported by policy recommendations:

1. *Create active societies. Create a paradigm shift in all of society by enhancing knowledge and understanding of, and appreciation for, the multiple benefits of regular physical activity, according to ability and at all ages, by changing social norms and attitudes around physical activity.* "We won't get the environmental changes and transport changes unless we get a shift in priority that walking and cycling is important, that green space is important."
2. *Create active environments. Create and maintain environments that promote and safeguard the rights of all people, of all ages, to have equitable access to safe places and spaces, in their cities and communities, in which to engage in regular physical activity, according to ability.* In cities and towns, there are differences in the opportunities for safe places for physical activity. Traffic congestion and road safety issues abound in some places where walking and cycling are promoted, and cross-sector partnerships can address some of these issues.
3. *Create active people. Create and promote access to opportunities and programs, across multiple settings, to help people of all ages*

and abilities to engage in regular physical activity as individuals, families, and communities.
4. *Create active systems. Create and strengthen leadership, governance, multisectoral partnerships, workforce capabilities, and advocacy and information systems across sectors to achieve excellence in resource mobilization and implementation of coordinated international, national, and subnational action.*

Taken together in a systems approach, Bull argued, these four objectives and their supporting strategies are interconnected and mutually supporting.

Bull went on to report that dissemination of WHO's plan and its call for multisector commitment and action is occurring through a global launch, regional launches, webinars, national events, and stakeholder forums and conferences. She emphasized the importance of tailored, region-specific tools that combine evidence, rationale, and practice examples to make progress in implementation. She elaborated that countries need resources and "how to" guides for developing or updating their national action plans for physical activity, conducting communication and social marketing campaigns, integrating physical activity into the guidance patients receive from health and social care services, and promoting physical activity in schools. She stressed that countries also need help with capacity building for multisector collaboration, and noted the challenges of bringing government departments together to build a "whole-of-system" approach. She added that monitoring and evaluation are important for holding countries accountable for their progress in implementing their action plans. To that end, she explained, a global monitoring framework will track indicators and metrics with which to gauge success in achieving the WHO plan's four strategic objectives.

Bull closed with a brief discussion of how physical activity policies can, both directly and indirectly, help achieve the United Nations' 17 Sustainable Development Goals. She underscored that creating a more active society cannot be achieved by the health sector alone; rather, working together across sectors is imperative, from the national to the local level.

FOOD AND NUTRITION INITIATIVES IN LATIN AMERICA AND THE CARIBBEAN

Fabio da Silva Gomes, regional advisor on nutrition and physical activity for the Americas, Pan American Health Organization/WHO, discussed food and nutrition actions taken by Latin America and the Caribbean to support obesity solutions. He cited as a lesson learned from the region's experience that it is common to jump from problems to solutions "without digging into the causes." He emphasized, however, that "the causes are probably where we can find most of the solutions," and he invited the workshop participants to think through the causes that introduce and promote obesity and undermine its solutions. One way to learn from the causes and devise solutions, he suggested, is to "think on the opposite side" by identifying approaches to worsen diets and expand obesity.

Pointing out that eating ultraprocessed foods[1] is associated with poorer dietary quality and higher obesity prevalence, da Silva Gomes emphasized that "there is no population that eats more ultraprocessed products and eats better." He displayed a series of graphs showing that in various countries, a greater proportion of energy intake from ultraprocessed products is correlated with a higher intake of sugars and saturated fat and lower intake of fiber (Cediel et al., 2018; Cornwell et al., 2018; Costa Louzada et al., 2015; Julia et al., 2018; Juul and Hemmingsson, 2015; Martinez-Steel et al., 2016; Monteiro et al., 2018). He explained further that the non-nutrient profile of these foods is obesity promoting, with characteristics that encourage faster consumption (such as being easy to chew, crush, and cut), slower and weaker satiety, and less compensation from other energy sources (Fardet, 2016; Fardet et al., 2017, 2018; Gombi-Vaca et al., 2016). He pointed to ecological data indicating that greater annual per capita retail sales of ultraprocessed products (in kilograms) and greater household relative availability of these foods in the Americas and in Europe, respectively, are associated with higher obesity prevalence (Monteiro et al., 2018; PAHO, 2015).

On the other hand, da Silva Gomes continued, "real food" is not a good choice to promote obesity because its lower energy density means that people would need to eat much greater quantities. Such food also takes more time to prepare and eat, he observed, and requires sitting down to eat rather than eating while multitasking. The "Golden Rule," he stated, is to always prefer natural or minimally processed foods and freshly made dishes and meals over ultraprocessed products (e.g., Ministry of Health of Brazil, 2015). He added that obesity will not be solved solely by promoting real food or by reducing the calories in ultraprocessed products. He argued for regulation of ultraprocessed products, and he again invited participants to take a counterapproach by asking, What are policies and practices that would promote excessive consumption of these foods?

In response to this question, da Silva Gomes stated that a solution to promote obesity is to use advertising and marketing to promote the consumption of ultraprocessed products. He briefly cited evidence demonstrat-

---

[1] The Pan American Health Organization defines "ultraprocessed foods" as industrial formulations manufactured from substances derived from foods or synthesized from other organic sources. See http://iris.paho.org/xmlui/bitstream/handle/123456789/7699/9789275118641_eng.pdf (accessed December 27, 2018).

ing the positive effect of advertising and marketing on sales (Assmus et al., 1984; Davis and Carpenter, 2009; Kelly et al., 2010; Woodside and Waddle, 1975), including the use of licensed characters and other front-of-package labeling techniques. To illustrate this point, he cited the sensation transfer theory, according to which children rate products as better tasting when popular media characters are on the packaging (Lapierre et al., 2011). He added that ultraprocessed products may be advertised to suggest a particular way of eating. As an example, he pointed to a chocolate product with a name that translates to "nonstop," remarking that this name suggests consuming the product compulsively. Thus, he asserted, regulation of advertising and marketing is necessary to help solve obesity. He referenced the example of Chile's front-of-package warning labels that alert consumers to a high amount of saturated fat or added sugars. Products that carry the warning labels cannot use licensed characters, are banned from schools, and are restricted as to how they are advertised (e.g., using toys).

Stressing that the relative affordability of ultraprocessed products contributes to their displacement of "real foods," da Silva Gomes advocated for correcting the distortion of prices so that real foods are more affordable, and ultraprocessed products are less affordable. He also encouraged clear, straightforward front-of-package labeling, citing data demonstrating that consumers try to minimize cognitive effort in repeat in-store purchasing decisions (Hoyer, 1984).

Lastly, da Silva Gomes described how solutions are undermined in the region by the opposition's efforts to weaken, delay, or impede them. "Part of the solution," he asserted, "is exposing and studying these tactics that corporations are using to push back the solutions." For instance, he said, these entities try to weaken or delay legislation, even resorting to legal tactics. Another tactic, he observed, is to shape the evidence base and frame the debate on diet- and public health–related issues. He shared a review paper comparing scientific studies funded by industry and nonindustry sources, noting that the industry-funded studies were more likely to report favorable conclusions, even if their results were unfavorable (Mandrioli et al., 2016). He cautioned that disclosure of conflict of interest is insufficient, declaring that "it actually can generate a sensation that you are now free to say whatever you want and to favor other results," and noting that some researchers fail to declare industry ties (e.g., Serodio et al., 2018). Finally, he briefly mentioned a press article describing one large company's efforts to monitor its reputation in social media (Thomasson, 2012), claiming that one of the company's purposes is to curb the spread of content that may jeopardize its credibility.

In closing, da Silva Gomes emphasized that it is important not only to expose the problems, but also to show that it is possible to do things differently.

DISCUSSION

During a discussion period following the three presentations summarized above, speakers shared examples of strategies for reducing disparities related to obesity prevalence, dietary intake, and physical activity patterns. Speakers also elaborated on physical activity, discussing its incorporation into health care counseling and its relationship to obesity prevalence.

Barata Cavalcanti urged an attitude of humility in order to "understand that we have quite a few things to learn from low-income countries," and called for increased sharing of data and information among countries. Bull asserted that disaggregated data, stratified beyond age and gender, could provide unique insights to help in crafting solutions. She described initiatives in Buenos Aires and London to collect suburb-level data on physical activity levels, as well as the environmental factors that affect physical activity. She pointed out that those data have helped these cities move from identifying the problem to developing tailored interventions to target the least active people in various suburbs. It was suggested by da Silva Gomes that school meals programs could improve students' diet quality and leverage local economies and agrobiodiversity by sourcing 30 percent of foods from local sources. This approach, he added, would favor indigenous populations and other traditional people who produce fruits and vegetables.

Health Care

In response to a participant's question about whether national health care systems are implementing physical activity counseling, Barata Cavalcanti responded that this intervention had not been highlighted by the MAPPS program's key informants. "Physical activity was very much at the bottom of the priorities for countries, unfortunately," she relayed. Bull concurred, saying that "it is a sad state," and noting that patients do not consistently receive physical activity advice from health care systems or health care providers, despite this being a recommended intervention. "There are examples of countries doing things," she acknowledged, "but we want to scale the very best practice and tailor it to all countries. It is a major priority for the health system."

Another participant observed that obesity treatment is often overshadowed by a focus on prevention, and wondered whether this is because treatment is generally not as available. She asked Barata Cavalcanti what types of treatment countries offer and whether the World Obesity Federation recommends specific offerings for different health systems based on their capacities and resources. Barata Cavalcanti replied that treatment is usually a combination of access to surgery and standardized medication, along with nutritional counseling. However, she observed, the advertised treatments are not always available in reality. As an example, she cited the availability of bariatric surgery in Brazil to individuals who meet prerequisites. But according to MAPPS key informants, she reported, "the waiting list is so long that you would have to wait around 100 years to get your surgery." She added that the World Obesity Federation will try to clarify what treatments are actually available in practice, and noted that while it is not yet making recommendations to health care systems, any guidance would feature a multidisciplinary team approach.

Bull responded to a participant's question about whether an association has been observed between physical inactivity and obesity across countries. She pointed to considerable variability in physical activity levels among, within, and across countries by gender. "The differences can reach up to 20 percent," she added, "which is quite substantial." She stated further that, although the data on the prevalence of physical inactivity and obesity could be graphed together, it is her belief that a positive association exists. She encouraged the workshop participants to keep in mind that physical activity can be integrated into the day in small ways, and encouraged framing activity as an enjoyable alternative to sedentary behaviors and entertainment. "We have to bring the fun back into it," she urged.

4

Managing the Global Epidemic: Challenges and Cross-Cultural Insights

> **Highlights from the Presentations of Individual Speakers**
>
> - Initiatives such as a soda tax and front-of-package warning labels have been implemented to help prevent and control obesity in Latin America, but these and other related efforts have been influenced by multinational food and beverage companies. (Simón Barquera)
> - Obesity is more prevalent in ethnic minority and migrant populations than in reference or host populations, and pathways emanating from social stratification based on race or ethnicity are implicated. Thus, disrupting racism and other discriminatory ideologies ("isms") and addressing these populations' historical and ongoing stressors may be critical to effective solutions. (Shiriki Kumanyika)
> - Indigenous Peoples' food systems and practices can inform solutions to the global obesity epidemic. Cultivating self-determination is key to preventing obesity in Indigenous populations, as is understanding the ecology and the environment in their home territories. (Harriet Kuhnlein)

Rachel Nugent, vice president for noncommunicable diseases (NCDs) at RTI International, returned to moderate the workshop's third session. In this session, three speakers explored in greater depth the challenges and cross-cultural insights associated with efforts to prevent and control obesity.

NAVIGATING THE OBESITY EPIDEMIC: THE MEXICO EXPERIENCE

Simón Barquera, director of the Nutrition and Health Research Center at the Mexican National Institute of Public Health, discussed some of the challenges associated with Mexico's efforts to prevent and control obesity. He noted that the country's prevalence of overweight and obesity has been increasing since measurement began in 1999, and is currently at nearly 73 percent. Relatedly, he observed, Mexico's mortality attributable to diabetes (9.34 percent) is among the highest in the world (GBD 2013 Mortality and Causes of Death Collaborators, 2015). In 2016, the Mexican government declared the diabetes epidemic a national health emergency, he said, explaining that this epidemiological alert was the first one Mexico had issued for an NCD.

Barquera highlighted what he characterized as successful initiatives to help prevent and control obesity in Latin America, including a soda tax implemented in Mexico in 2014 and later in Chile, Ecuador, and Peru. He cited evaluation data for Mexico's soda tax showing a reduction in purchases of sugar-sweetened beverages that was sustained 2 years after the tax had been implemented and averaged 7.6 percent (Colchero et al., 2017). This may sound like a small effect, he observed, "but in a country of 126 million inhabitants, this represents about 67,000 tons of sugar that were not consumed in these 2 years." Mexico's soda tax model has been used in other countries, he added, and it will continue to be refined. He also highlighted contrasts in the packaging of the same cereal product in Mexico and in Chile, noting that Chile has stricter front-of-package regulations.

Barquera cited several challenges for obesity prevention efforts in Latin America: the presence of the double burden of malnutrition and inequalities in obesity prevalence associated with socioeconomic status (see Chapter 2), scarce resources to invest in obesity prevention and in evaluation of interventions, and primary health care systems that were created when infectious diseases were the main concern and thus lack the resources to handle chronic diseases.

Barquera highlighted as another challenge that Mexico experiences interference from industry, such as aggressive marketing of unhealthy foods in poor communities. He pointed out that healthy foods such as fruits and vegetables are inexpensive in Mexico, so to sell junk foods and soft drinks, Mexican companies are more aggressive than those in other nations. He cited results of an evaluation in five countries that found point-of-purchase advertisements directed at children in a higher proportion of low-income than high-income stores. These type of advertisements are common, he observed, and include cartoon characters on packages, price discounts, and free gifts. And they work, he noted, because sugar-sweetened beverages

MANAGING THE GLOBAL EPIDEMIC 43

and sweet and salty snacks are the top products customers reported buying without prior planning.

Considering opportunities in obesity prevention in Latin America, Barquera explained that the obesity problem has high political visibility in the region. He explained that close connections among the region's countries have led to a domino effect for some policies as countries have consulted with each other. Because many cost-effective interventions to prevent obesity do not involve expensive technology, he added, they can be replicated in low- and middle-income countries worldwide.

Barquera then shifted his attention to front-of-package nutrition labels as a strategy for helping consumers make healthier food choices. He contrasted the Guideline Daily Amount (GDA) label system developed by the food industry in Mexico with Chile's warning label system, which was developed by academics (see Figure 4-1).

The GDA label is complex, misleading, and difficult to interpret in making food decisions, Barquera argued. He cited research suggesting that this label is not well understood by Mexican nutrition students at the university level (Stern et al., 2011), and that only 13.8 percent of respondents in a Mexican national survey said they understood it. In a multinational survey of high-income populations, 54 percent responded that they understood the GDA label, while 83 percent responded that they understood the warning label, he reported. That study also found that lower-income populations had a lower probability of understanding and using the GDAs to make healthier choices, he added. The warning label is easily interpreted,

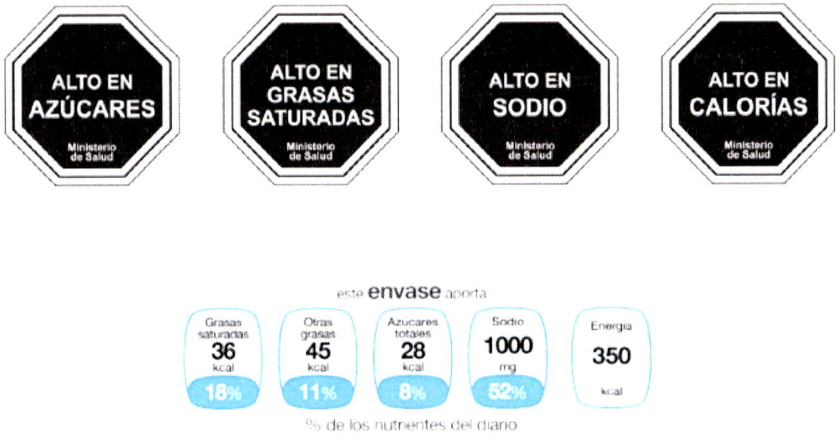

FIGURE 4-1 Warning label system implemented in Chile (top) and Guideline Daily Amount label system implemented in Mexico (bottom).
SOURCE: Presented by Simón Barquera, October 9, 2018.

he argued. "In Chile, even the kids know that when they have this octagon, it means that there is something wrong with the product. It's high in something."

Barquera then turned to the Mexican Observatory for Obesity, describing it as a government-appointed advisory council that makes decisions about obesity prevention actions in Mexico. About half of the council members are associated with the food industry, he said, adding that these members opposed public health and obesity prevention initiatives that were submitted to the council. He stated that he and his colleagues have tried to expose this coordinated response of opposition by publishing evaluations of "how the process goes when you have this kind of interference from industry" (Barquera et al., 2018).

The Mexican National Institute of Public Health convened what Barquera called a "conflict of interest–free" group of academics to make evidence-based recommendations for front-of-package labeling. The group observed that the GDA label is not an effective system for promoting healthier choices, he reported, and it suggested that a front-of-package label could be simple and based on established national or international nutrition standards. Barquera noted that the group's report will be presented to Mexico's incoming national political administration.

Barquera moved on to describe the Mexican health system's lack of capacity for obesity prevention and control. The country's total health budget is relatively low, he observed, and he characterized the proportion of the budget dedicated to chronic disease prevention as inadequate (Barquera and White, 2018). He asserted further that physicians are not adequately trained to screen for and treat obesity, and there are not enough specialists to whom patients can be referred. He argued that major adjustments in the budget and in the organization of health services could control the spread of obesity with effective treatment.

Barquera ended by calling for (1) the promotion of "double-duty policies" that can affect both undernutrition and obesity, with a focus on groups of low socioeconomic status (see Chapter 2); (2) refinement of tax policies and implementation of other regulations to improve obesogenic environments; and (3) mitigation of industry interference, particularly from multinational companies, in the decision-making parts of the system. "We need to speak out about this," he concluded, "because many of these companies say they want to be part of the solution in international meetings . . . but at the local level, they are really part of the problem and they are not willing to accept any type of regulation or attempt of the government to improve the environment."

COMMON THREADS IN OBESITY RISK AMONG RACIAL/ETHNIC AND MIGRANT MINORITY POPULATIONS

Shiriki Kumanyika, research professor in the Department of Community Health and Prevention, Drexel Dornsife School of Public Health, Drexel University, and emeritus professor of epidemiology, Perelman School of Medicine, University of Pennsylvania, shared cross-cultural insights about populations at above-average risk for obesity within high-income countries.

Kumanyika took a health inequities perspective in her presentation, exploring common threads in obesity risk among racial/ethnic and migrant minority populations. Pointing out that racial/ethnic minority status is associated with above-average obesity risk compared with white majority populations, she asserted that examining patterns of obesity risk in populations of color in different country contexts can lead to new insights and potentially to solutions (Kumanyika et al., 2012). For context, she noted that population-wide increases in obesity are driven by societal forces—and the policies governing them—that relate directly or indirectly to food systems or physical activity and converge to make it difficult for people to control their weight. Apparently, she continued, within high-income countries these forces operate differentially for minority populations, and the question is why.

Kumanyika went on to review data on obesity prevalence stratified by racial/ethnic group for adults in Australia, England, the Netherlands, New Zealand, and the United States (Australian Bureau of Statistics, 2013; CDC, 2016; Hales et al., 2017; New Zealand Ministry of Health, 2018; Public Health England, 2016; Schmengler et al., 2017). She highlighted a tendency toward higher obesity prevalence in minority populations of color relative to reference or host populations in these countries, especially among women. She also flagged the lower prevalence of obesity in Asian populations in these countries and reminded the audience that the data are based on a body mass index (BMI) cutoff of 30. Referencing the discussion of ethnic-specific BMI cutoffs in session 1 of the workshop (see Chapter 2), she expressed concern about the continued use of this cutoff for obesity in Asian populations, arguing that it will yield "an answer that's misleading in terms of health risk."

Kumanyika proceeded to observe that, according to longitudinal studies, migrants' lower weights yield to excess weight gain over time. This phenomenon is sometimes attributed to acculturation or studied as a matter of duration of residence in the host country, she noted, adding that cross-national studies within these ethnic groups point to effects of Western environments compared with the environments in migrants' countries of origin. "These data have been critical to refute the idea of default genetic explanations," she explained, because the finding that people with the same general genetic background have higher weights when living in different circumstances suggests a role for nongenetic (i.e., environmental) factors. Accordingly, she observed, environmental explanations now dominate the discussion. She added that cross-national studies within Western environments indicate effects of national contexts, and she reminded participants of Meeks's data on the differences among Ghanaian populations living in three European cities (see Chapter 2).

Kumanyika went on to identify one key question to consider: What is different about minority populations of color compared with host or reference populations? She then cited a second key question: What is similar in different societies with respect to minority populations of color? She noted that these questions are important to explore for children as well as adults but are much more complex, pointing out that in children, one must account for weight gain patterns during growth and development in relation to age at migration, among other factors.

Kumanyika paused to consider historical aspects of the collection of data on race and ethnicity. She suggested that when such data are collected, the implication is that the data have societal importance, such as relevance for policy making. She pointed out that the collection of racial and ethnic data is routine in the United States, although the categories used in the research evolve. In contrast, she said, Europe has in the past been reluctant to collect data on residents' ethnicity, preferring "color blindness" and distinguishing health inequities by social class (Loring and Robertson, 2014; Simon, 2012). She noted, however, a recent movement toward collecting racial and ethnic data based on their importance to health policy.

Kumanyika then referenced a World Health Organization (WHO) Commission report on ending childhood obesity (2016b), which makes the point that effects of socioeconomic status in high-income countries differ from those in low- and middle-income countries. In high-income countries, she explained, risks of childhood obesity are greatest among groups of lower socioeconomic status, but the converse is true in most low- and middle-income countries, although these patterns are becoming more complex. Within high-income countries, certain population subgroups (such as migrant and indigenous children) are at particularly high risk of obesity, she elaborated, which the WHO report attributes to rapid acculturation and poor access to public health information. However, Kumanyika emphasized that these two factors are only a part of the story of how environmental factors operate differentially in these subgroups.

Kumanyika then turned her attention to potential influences on obesity in minority populations of color (which include migrant groups), citing the following variables: racial/ethnic category, socioeconomic status and social position, migration and migration stress, language and literacy, cultural assets, structural empowerment and resilience, and stress. For each set of variables, she discussed the associated contextual factors that might influence weight (see Table 4-1). She pointed out that although stress is listed separately, it is highlighted because its influence is moderated through pathways related to all of the other variables.

Finally, Kumanyika described her framework for depicting pathways that produce racial/ethnic and migrant inequities in obesity, along with potential intervention points (see Figure 4-2). She hypothesized an intersection among race/ethnicity, migrant status, and any other stratification

TABLE 4-1 Potential Influences on Obesity in Minority Populations of Color

Variable	Contexts
Racial/ethnic category (explicit or implicit, i.e., not being white)	• Cultural food preferences • Neighborhood access (segregation) • Targeted marketing of unhealthy foods • Mobility (freedom of movement) • Historical and ongoing trauma
Socioeconomic status; social position	• Neighborhood access (poverty) • Food purchasing power • Activity patterns • Housing • Access to health care
Migration and migration stress	• Adverse circumstances prior to or during migration • Abrupt exposure to obesogenic environment • Loss of connections with home environment • Downward mobility
Language/literacy	• Access to nutrition information • Access to quality education • Better social integration
Cultural assets and protection	• Preservation of traditional healthy behaviors • Buffering from aggressive promotion of unhealthy foods and beverages • Coping mechanisms, including faith
Structural empowerment and resilience	• Ability to benefit from new opportunities • Social capital and social support
Stress	• Eating and physical activity • "Embodiment" • Constant need to cope • Sleep

NOTE: Stress is highlighted to denote that its influence is moderated through pathways related to all of the other variables.
SOURCES: Adapted from Kumanyika, 2018. Presented by Shiriki Kumanyika, October 9, 2018.

variables that apply in a country to determine health inequities, as outlined in the WHO conceptual framework for action on the social determinants of health (Solar and Irwin, 2010). These inequities, she explained, then condition the social determinants of health (such as neighborhood of residence and access to health care).

Kumanyika ended by reiterating that obesity is often more prevalent in racial and ethnic minorities and migrants versus reference or host populations, and that race/ethnicity and migration intersect. She suggested that studying these patterns in diverse high-income countries could yield new insights to inform policy actions. She challenged the audience to consider that "if the pathways arise solely or in part from social stratification, then the ultimate solutions to this excess risk in populations of color require a major disruption in the 'isms' that got [us to] where we are today."

THE CONTRIBUTION OF TRADITIONAL CULTURES TO RESOLVING THE OBESITY PANDEMIC

Harriet Kuhnlein, emerita professor at McGill University, focused on Indigenous Peoples as she explored how traditional cultures can inform solutions for the obesity pandemic. Although many countries lack census data disaggregated by ethnicity, she began, the United Nations has on record 370 million Indigenous and tribal people in more than 90 countries, repre-

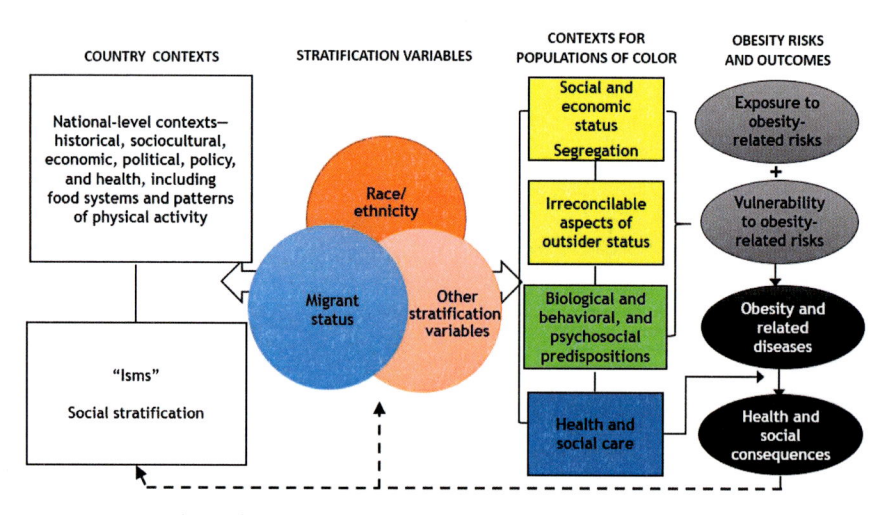

FIGURE 4-2 Pathway for production of racial/ethnic and migrant inequities in obesity and potential points to intervene.
SOURCES: Adapted from Kumanyika, 2018. Presented by Shiriki Kumanyika, October 9, 2018.

senting 5,000 identified groups and about 4,000 languages. These people are among the poorest in the world, she observed, and face intractable poverty, racism, and discrimination. They also have lower life expectancy; less access to education, employment, and standard housing; and more violence and incarceration. The United Nations has recognized that their marginalization is due to violation of their right to traditional lands and territories, Kuhnlein added (UN, 2009, 2013, 2017b).

According to Kuhnlein, researchers look to Indigenous Peoples in rural areas to gain insights as to what their food systems might offer in terms of obesity solutions because of their connectedness to nature. They have inhabited their territories for long periods of time, she elaborated, so they have been sustainable with their food systems. And based on the limited information available, she added, "we recognize that most of these people were not obese." Indigenous Peoples' knowledge of food systems is derived from their collective experience in managing 22 percent of the world's ecosystems and land mass, she explained, as well as understanding the planet's animal and plant natural resources and preserving much of its biodiversity (Burlingame and Dernini, 2019).

Kuhnlein described a study of the local food resources of 12 cultures, reporting that the researchers discovered unique and delicious foods with surprising nutrient values. They tallied the number of species used as food in each culture, finding that it reached nearly 400 in some tropical locations. Based on dietary records collected in the field, Kuhnlein noted, those traditional local foods represented anywhere from 10 to 98 percent of the energy consumed by people in these 12 cultures (Kuhnlein et al., 2009). The researchers also learned how those foods are being lost to global agricultural and food marketing practices (Kuhnlein et al., 2009, 2013).

Kuhnlein stressed that the loss of indigenous food system knowledge poses a number of risks. Those risks include habitat destruction and ecosystem threats such as resource (e.g., oil) extraction, land grabs, and climate change, in addition to displacement from indigenous territory, loss of language and culture, urbanization and migration of knowledge holders and youth, acceptance of more commercial foods, and loss of seeds and wildlife (Kuhnlein et al., 2009, 2013; UN, 2009, 2013, 2017b).

Kuhnlein then transitioned to discuss current statistics on obesity and stunting among Indigenous Peoples. Citing data from the Centers for Disease Control and Prevention (CDC), she stated that nearly 75 percent of American Indian and Alaska Native adults have overweight or obesity, compared with about 61 percent of non-Hispanic white adults (CDC, 2017b). However, the prevalence of diabetes among these adult indigenous peoples is more than double that among their non-Hispanic white counterparts (17.6 versus 7.3 percent), she pointed out (CDC, 2010). She added that the figures for adolescent overweight and obesity are similar for indigenous populations and non-Hispanic whites, and suggested further research to track when those numbers diverge. Turning to undernutrition, she referenced census and health data from Brazil, Colombia, India, and Peru, revealing that the prevalence of stunting in children less than 5 years of age is much greater among indigenous populations than benchmark populations in each country (Anderson et al., 2016).

Kuhnlein asserted that a systems approach is key to preventing obesity in Indigenous Peoples, as is understanding the ecology and the environment in their home territories. She highlighted self-determination as an element that can lead to sustainable food systems, food security, and health. To build capacity for self-determination, she called for using community-specific information as a platform for health promotion activities; respecting indigenous ways of knowing and being; and recognizing the "global megaforces" that undermine Indigenous cultures, as well as the historical trauma that those cultures have experienced. She also stressed the importance of helping these communities understand the nutrient composition of their foods and the impact of a transition to commercial foods. At the same time, however, she cautioned that "the impact of our education and awareness can be swamped out by the larger ecological factors such as poverty or food access."

Kuhnlein then shared Lemke and Delormier's (2017) views on how to meet the challenges of obesity in Indigenous Peoples: (1) decolonize public health programs to express holistic worldviews to prevent obesity and undernutrition; (2) use the Indigenous values of respect, responsibilities, and relationships to each other and to nature; (3) recognize locally specific conditions and the broader historical, political, cultural, economic, and environmental contexts; and (4) build the indigenous public health workforce to promote well-being based on human rights, and rebuild cultural morale with local practices.

According to Kuhnlein, Indigenous Peoples' experience can inform strategies for combating the obesity epidemic to the extent that researchers document and learn from their health strategies and the diversity of their food systems. "Indigenous Peoples understand that food use touches everything," she remarked, including mental, physical, social, and spiritual well-being. She proposed building an international platform for gathering knowledge of traditional and Indigenous holistic food systems and health systems with ecological sustainability, and urged intercultural education as a way to help resolve the obesity pandemic.

DISCUSSION

A brief discussion period followed this third session of the workshop. Topics included co-creation of strategies for addressing obesity in minority populations of color, acculturation, building an international knowledge platform, and globalization and global megaforces.

Co-Creation of Strategies for Addressing Obesity

A participant observed that the influences on obesity in minority populations, as outlined by Kumanyika, are serious problems in and of themselves. She asked Kumanyika how to ensure that these populations consider obesity a priority. Kumanyika suggested engaging with a community and learning about its members' priorities to build on their "insider knowledge and experience" in devising a sustainable solution, co-created with community members. This does not necessarily mean starting from the beginning and ignoring the interventions already developed, she clarified. However, she said, trying to just tweak an existing intervention to fit the community is too superficial, "so the movement toward co-creation could probably open some new doors."

Acculturation

Acculturation is a survival strategy for most populations that are migrating, a participant stated. She asked whether factors exist that are typically positive or negative with regard to obesity that are present as migrants acculturate. Kumanyika replied that both positives and negatives are related to the acculturation process, but suggested that it is problematic to use acculturation as the primary explanation for high obesity risk. A singular focus on acculturation, which is common, she elaborated, places the emphasis on how migrants are reacting without looking at how they are viewed and treated in the society. According to Kumanyika, acculturation implies that people may attempt, sometimes seemingly "against all odds," to integrate into a community, but what she termed their "irreconcilable outsider status" can make those attempts counterproductive in some respects. She proposed that it may be more productive for people to retain their cultural group perspectives and leverage the associated strengths, but acknowledged that the topic is extremely complex.

Kuhnlein recounted her experience broaching the topic of obesity with Indigenous Peoples in British Columbia. She recalled that they asked, "Oh, you want to deculturize us?" She emphasized the importance of allowing people to recognize their strengths and find solutions from within those strengths.

Building an International Knowledge Platform

A participant asked Kuhnlein to elaborate on her suggestion about building an international knowledge platform. Kuhnlein replied that some cultures want to handle obesity in their own way, while others are more interested in learning from others. In any case, she suggested that the many ideas about promoting consumption of healthy food are worth documenting, and noted that the Food and Agriculture Organization is building a platform to record Indigenous experiences.

Globalization and Global Megaforces

The impact of globalization on food and physical activity patterns throughout the world is apparent, observed a participant. He asked what Indigenous Peoples can teach others about how to decolonize from the globalized food economy. Kuhnlein agreed that Indigenous Peoples can offer wisdom about how to effect change within their own communities. She advised public health practitioners to conduct formative research in communities of interest, arguing that doing so is useful for building a good public health promotion program.

Nugent asked Barquera to elaborate on how Mexico is handling global mega-forces in its local obesity prevention efforts. Barquera replied that, because Mexico is a large market, lobbying efforts to oppose public health policies have been strong. As an example of how globalization of trade has impacted obesity prevention efforts, he cited the recent negotiation of a global trade agreement in North America, which included an attempt to limit countries' power to require warning labels on food products. This attempt was ultimately defeated, he noted, because public health and civil society groups spoke up. He added that countries with smaller economies may not experience as much opposition from multinational companies, and thus may have an easier time implementing regulations.

5

Reflections on the Global Approach and Lessons for Next Steps

> **Highlights from the Presentations of Individual Speakers**
> - Numerous and diverse strategies for promoting physical activity have been implemented around the world, but few have been evaluated. Many of these strategies could be adapted, implemented, and evaluated in the United States. (James Sallis)
> - Bloomberg Philanthropies works with leading advocacy and research organizations to raise awareness of obesity and to identify, implement, and evaluate effective obesity prevention policies in low- and middle-income countries. Through these activities, the organization hopes to accelerate the growth of the evidence base for obesity prevention strategies. (Neena Prasad)
> - Awareness of the obesity problem is increasing around the world, but concrete action at scale remains elusive. In addition to contributing money, the World Bank can use its convening power to gather high-level national leaders and ministries of finance to discuss solutions. (Meera Shekar)
> - Given the interrelationships among undernutrition, obesity, and climate change, stakeholders are urged to consider whether today's decisions will preserve the health of the planet and the health of the population several generations into the future. (Bill Dietz)

Speakers in the workshop's final session reflected on progress to date in addressing the obesity pandemic and discussed the lessons for obesity prevention and treatment efforts in the United States, especially with respect to reducing disparities. Bill Dietz, chair of the Sumner M. Redstone Global Center for Prevention and Wellness, Milken Institute School of Public Health, The George Washington University, moderated the session. He mentioned that the workshop planning committee thought it important for this session to revisit physical activity, and for it to include representatives from organizations that fund prevention and treatment efforts.

GLOBAL LESSONS FOR PHYSICAL ACTIVITY PROMOTION IN THE UNITED STATES

James Sallis, distinguished professor emeritus of family medicine and public health at the University of California, San Diego, and professorial fellow at the Australian Catholic University, Melbourne, described global lessons for physical activity promotion in the United States. He began with a brief overview of disparities in prevalence, environments, and policies with respect to physical activity in the United States, displaying data on the differences among four ethnic groups in walking for transportation and leisure (see Figure 5-1). Few differences exist in walking for transport,

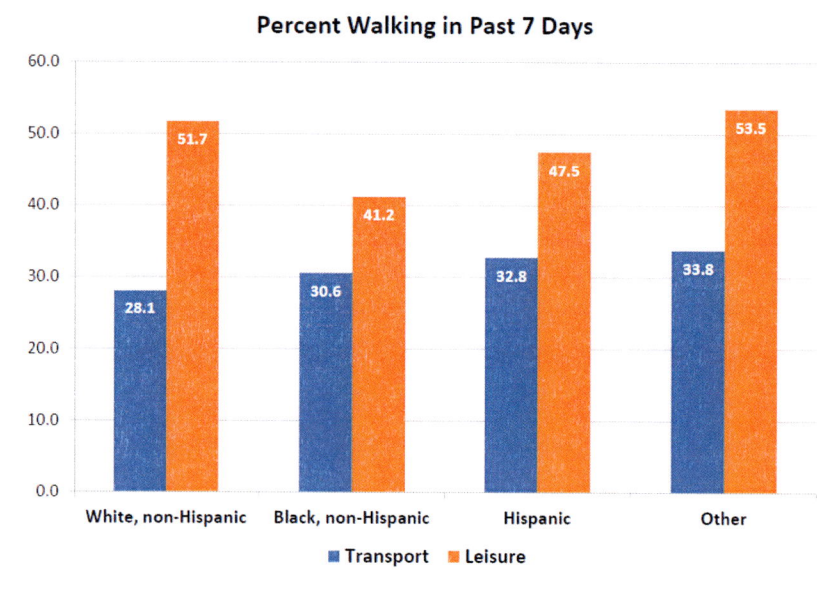

Percent Walking in Past 7 Days

Race/Ethnicity	Transport	Leisure
White, non-Hispanic	28.1	51.7
Black, non-Hispanic	30.6	41.2
Hispanic	32.8	47.5
Other	33.8	53.5

FIGURE 5-1 Walking for transportation and leisure: differences by race/ethnicity.
SOURCES: Adapted from Paul et al., 2015. Presented by James Sallis, October 9, 2018.

he remarked, but there are bigger differences in walking for leisure, with particularly lower levels among African Americans and Latinos. "Those are the disparities to pay attention to," he urged.

Sallis declared that disparities in the "activity friendliness" of U.S. environments are location-specific. "It's not one pattern across the country; it depends on where you are in the country," he explained. He stressed that it is essential to have local data to understand disparities in the quality of environments in a particular city. There may also be disparities in policy implementation, he added, citing a study of differences in the implementation of federally funded bicycle and pedestrian projects. The study found that counties in the United States with persistent poverty or low educational status were less likely to obtain funding for or to implement such projects (Cradock et al., 2009).

Next, Sallis shared a series of international examples of physical activity initiatives that he said could "inspire and instruct us." He provided examples for each of the four strategic objectives in the World Health Organization (WHO) Global Action Plan on Physical Activity.

Sallis first described ciclovias, "open street" practices aimed at creating active societies by closing miles of roads to cars and letting people take over the streets. Ciclovias were implemented in Bogotá, Colombia, for equity purposes, he explained, so that lower-income residents without cars could take advantage of the streets. This practice has become integrated into the culture in parts of Latin America, he observed, but in the United States is more limited in scope and frequency. "It's not a part of our culture," he observed. "It's a special event that nobody pays much attention to."

Next Sallis mentioned Brazil's "academias de saude," or "health academies," which facilitate and encourage physical activity in public spaces. "In my mind," he said, "that is creating a more active society, where everybody sees everybody else being active." However, he added, organized physical activity in public spaces is "something that we don't do very well here," and he called attention to a journal supplement focused on reports and evaluations of those efforts in other countries (Giles-Corti et al., 2017).

Turning to the strategy of creating active environments, Sallis reported that Spain has banned cars from some city centers. "For me, this is paradise," he quoted a resident of one of these cities saying in a newspaper headline. He encouraged making cities more bikable, noting that while 50 percent of all trips in the United States are bikable distances (up to 4 to 5 miles), the actual bike share of trips in cities is only 1 percent. He pointed to major cities around the world that have increased their bike share of trips through multilevel, multicomponent interventions over time (Pucher et al., 2010).

In the realm of creating active people, Sallis praised an enduring Canadian physical activity promotion initiative that began in 1971, called "ParticipACTION." Through a media campaign and public–private partnerships to promote its messages, he reported, its aim to change social norms about physical activity has coincided with Canada being one of the few countries with a trend of increasing physical activity. He also mentioned Agita Mundo, a Latin American initiative to "massively mobilize" people to become active, as well as Finland's requirement for 2 hours per day of physical activity in schools—"and they do better academically," he noted about the latter.

Sallis then pointed to the Thai Health Promotion Foundation as a sustainably funded example of creating active systems, explaining that it collects taxes on alcohol and tobacco to fund initiatives that promote healthy behaviors. As a second example, he cited South Africa's Bicycle Empowerment Network, which aims to alleviate poverty through promotion of bicycle use for commuting to jobs. According to data he shared from a recent study, lower-income households can save a considerable proportion of disposable income if they do not own cars and opt to use more active transport methods (Rachele et al., 2018).

Sallis closed by emphasizing that there are many good strategies for promoting physical activity around the world. He suggested that many of these strategies could be adapted, implemented, and evaluated in the United States given the necessary funding and political will for policy change.

PUBLIC POLICIES TO IMPROVE THE FOOD ENVIRONMENT

According to Neena Prasad, director of the global obesity prevention and maternal and reproductive health program at Bloomberg Philanthropies, her organization works with leading advocacy and research organizations to raise awareness of obesity and to identify, implement, and evaluate effective obesity prevention policies in six low- and middle-income countries: Barbados, Brazil, Colombia, Jamaica, Mexico, and South Africa. Bloomberg Philanthropies is also supporting the evaluation of marketing and front-of-package labeling policies in Chile and sugary beverage taxes in some U.S. cities through an Evaluation Fund, she added.

Prasad explained that the organization pursues national policy change in four priority areas—fiscal measures, marketing restrictions, front-of-package warning labels, and healthier schools—to improve food environments so that healthier options are the default. She added that these four priorities were chosen in consultation with leading scholars and are revisited regularly, although they have remained relatively consistent over the past 6 years. According to Prasad, the organization's largest investment is in tobacco control, and it is applying lessons from that arena to obesity prevention. "It's not a perfect parallel," she said, "but there are important similarities."

Bloomberg Philanthropies supports policy change by funding advocacy, mass media, and research activities, Prasad continued, and then evaluates policy implementation. To explain why the organization takes a regulatory approach, she contrasted rates of progress toward reducing consumption of sugary beverages for voluntary industry-coordinated initiatives and regulatory initiatives (Keybridge, 2018; Public Health England, 2018). The regulatory initiatives made a bigger impact in a shorter period of time, she reported. She emphasized her organization's commitment to evidence-based policy advocacy and shared examples of research that supports policy initiatives, such as modeling of the impact of a sugary beverage tax on diabetes and cardiovascular disease.

A large proportion of Bloomberg Philanthropies' resources goes toward public awareness campaigns, Prasad continued, which are usually coupled with policy campaigns. Based on the experience with tobacco control, she elaborated, "we tend to go for hard-hitting graphic campaigns." She shared an awareness-raising video that aired in conjunction with a sugary beverage tax campaign, reporting that pre- and posttesting indicated a positive impact on viewers' understanding of the causes and consequences of consuming sugary beverages, as well as their expectations of what their governments should be doing to protect them in this regard. Prasad asserted that grassroots activity and public buy-in are important because "often when policy makers know the public is on their side, they are more willing to take those risks" to support a policy campaign. In addition, she stressed, keeping an issue in the news and maintaining its sense of urgency creates and softens the ground for policy action.

Prasad went on to discuss Bloomberg Philanthropies' support for coalition-building activities, highlighting coalitions in South Africa, Brazil, and Mexico that she said have engaged numerous diverse, credible organizations to advocate for shared interests. If policy is instituted, she added, the organization supports evaluation postimplementation to assess its impact (e.g., Colchero et al., 2016, 2017; Guerrero-Lopez et al., 2017; Silver et al., 2017). She noted that after Mexico adopted a sugary drink tax in 2014, a number of other countries followed suit. "We are optimistic that this is soon going to become a public health norm," she said.

To wrap up, Prasad underscored that Bloomberg Philanthropies wants to accelerate the growth of the evidence base for "what works" in obesity prevention. She stated that the organization wants to achieve the implementation of diverse policies in its six focus countries, evaluate the early impact of policies in both its focus and nonfocus countries, and construct the beginnings of a policy package that any country can begin to adopt.

A PERSPECTIVE FROM THE WORLD BANK

The World Bank focuses on obesity as an economic issue, said Meera Shekar, global lead for nutrition with the World Bank's health, nutrition, and population global practice. She warned that it is only a matter of time before obesity overwhelms the health sector and the economy in countries across the globe, pointing out that the problem affects low-, middle-, and high-income countries. She also explained that as a country's per capita income increases, the burden of overweight and obesity shifts to the poor. Echoing the workshop's earlier discussion about the double burden (see Chapter 2), she noted that mapping a country's overweight and obesity alongside stunting helps determine which strategies to pursue.

Shekar briefly mentioned nine country case studies of health promotion strategies and policies that the World Bank is reviewing to determine scalability in different conditions. These include fiscal and regulatory policies, she said, as well as education, media, and transportation strategies and traditional nutrition interventions. She then highlighted key milestones in global action on obesity and previewed a number of forthcoming reports. However, many reports on noncommunicable diseases fail to focus on overweight and obesity, and "that's something I think we might try and fix," she noted.

The World Bank has invested considerable funding in efforts to address undernutrition, Shekar continued, but while awareness of the obesity problem is increasing, concrete action at scale in this area remains elusive. She suggested that while the World Bank contributes money, what is more useful is its power to convene high-level national leaders and decision makers, as well as ministries of finance, and reach them with messages and evidence. In addition, she maintained, mobilizing domestic resources is critical to change the financing landscape for any of these issues.

Shekar then turned to the World Bank's new Human Capital Project, which, she said, will accelerate more and better investments in people globally. She characterized this as a major shift from the World Bank's reputation as a "hard infrastructure bank." The project, she explained, will include a Human Capital Index to make the case for investment in the human capital of the next generation, focusing on health and education; improve measurement and provide analysis to support investments in human capital formation; and support early adopters, and ultimately all countries, in preparing national strategies that accelerate progress on human capital.

In closing, Shekar shared three ways for the World Bank to support obesity prevention and control efforts: maximize the potential of its multisectoral engagement (with the health, agriculture, transport, and fiscal sectors, for example); scale up promising policies and interventions; and leverage the range of World Bank instruments at all levels. At the global level, she elaborated, this might include advocating for the incorporation of obesity efforts into universal health care and poverty reduction efforts; at the country level, it might entail the use of policy instruments such as development policy operations. The latter initiatives come into play, she explained, when the World Bank enters into an agreement to release resources to a government if the country implements designated policies. Lastly, Shekar reiterated that there are many lessons to be learned from the tobacco control movement—particularly its taxation strategy—and highlighted building broad alliances.

TYING IT ALL TOGETHER

Reflecting on the day's presentations, session moderator Bill Dietz applauded what he called a rich series of talks that had covered many topics and themes. He made a number of observations:

- Trends in obesity prevalence are parallel for men and women and for developed and developing countries, suggesting that the exposures that led to obesity were simultaneously distributed across the population.
- Health systems will be challenged by obesity and an ensuing wave of diabetes.
- As they face rapid urbanization, low-income countries may need to advocate for preservation of their activity-promoting built environments.
- It is important to be aware that some cultures have social norms that value obesity or at least do not consider it a problem.
- The globalization of the U.S. food supply has contributed to the obesity epidemic, and it was suggested that the health sector continue to establish trust with the food industry if a positive difference in the healthfulness of the food supply is to be made. According to the workshop's presentations, it appears that a lack of trust between the two sectors is a bigger problem in Latin America than in the United States.
- It will not be possible to confront the racial and ethnic disparities in the development of obesity without confronting the inequities that lead to these disparities. Just as the consequences of adverse childhood experiences may not be fully expressed until adulthood, the consequences of these inequities may not manifest as disparities in obesity prevalence until later in life.

To conclude, Dietz maintained that sustainability is integral to the workshop's discussions, given the relationship between the agricultural production and distribution system and the emission of greenhouse gases, for example. He challenged participants to consider sustainability in light of the interrelationships among undernutrition, obesity, and climate change. He cited a decision-making practice of the Iroquois Confederacy, a group of several Native American tribes that controlled the northwest corner of the United States when the Europeans arrived. They considered how their decisions would affect people seven generations into the future, he said, and asked, "How do we ensure that our decisions are going to preserve the planet, planetary health, and the health of the population for the seventh generation?"

DISCUSSION

During the final discussion period, workshop participants considered the viability of fiscal strategies for helping to prevent and control obesity and the importance of evaluation.

Fiscal Strategies

Speakers touched on challenges and opportunities with respect to fiscal strategies for helping to address the obesity pandemic, such as taxes on unhealthy foods and financial incentives for healthy behaviors. Prasad said that although taxation is considered an effective strategy for tobacco control, her group has found discussion of earmarking of tax revenues for this purpose to be an unproductive conversation with ministries of finance. She pointed to promotion funds, such as the example from Thailand shared by Sallis, as another fiscal idea, one that is promising from a public health perspective. Shekar agreed that fiscal strategies can be promoted in conversations with ministries of finance, but urged the development of alternative, innovative financing sources. On that note, Sallis raised the idea of financial incentives for healthy behaviors such as walking or bicycling. He also suggested that health benefits could be realized if transportation budgets were reduced, quoting an economist from the Asian Development Bank who said that the cost to construct one freeway flyover could instead be used to build 800 miles of protected bike lanes. That would "revolutionize any city in this country, and one flyover would not be missed," Sallis claimed.

The Importance of Evaluation

Rigorous evaluation of programs and "natural experiments" such as policy change, attendees observed, are critical to understanding a theory's practical effectiveness and can help determine whether further investment in a particular strategy is worthwhile. One participant suggested that there may be surprises about the causal pathways for obesity, and Shekar reiterated that building evaluation into large-scale programming is critical. Prasad concurred and advocated for taking action based on the best available evidence rather than waiting to act. It is inevitable that there will be some mistakes, she conceded, but "we can't afford to wait to understand every aspect of this before we act." Sallis agreed and added that the available evidence may not be definitive, but it is good fodder for hypotheses that could be tested. He questioned whether there have been enough interventions of sufficient magnitude to effect lasting change, and asserted, "The more I look into this, the more I see that we need to stimulate bold action, and then evaluate it."

Bill Purcell concluded the workshop by stating that the Roundtable on Obesity Solutions will continue to explore the topic of global obesity and the implications for prevention and treatment efforts in the United States: "This is a conversation that we have been waiting to start for some time," he said, and "I think . . . we're at the beginning of that conversation."

References

Agyemang, C., E. Owusu-Dabo, A. de Jonge, D. Martins, G. Ogedegbe, and K. Stronks. 2009. Overweight and obesity among Ghanaian residents in the Netherlands: How do they weigh against their urban and rural counterparts in Ghana? *Public Health Nutrition* 12(7):909–916.

Agyemang, C., K. Stronks, N. Tromp, R. Bhopal, P. Zaninotto, N. Unwin, J. Nazroo, and A. E. Kunst. 2010. A cross-national comparative study of smoking prevalence and cessation between English and Dutch south Asian and African origin populations: The role of national context. *Nicotine & Tobacco Research: Official Journal of the Society for Research on Nicotine and Tobacco* 12(6):557–566.

Agyemang, C., K. Meeks, E. Beune, E. Owusu-Dabo, F. P. Mockenhaupt, J. Addo, A. de Graft Aikins, S. Bahendeka, I. Danquah, M. B. Schulze, J. Spranger, T. Burr, P. Agyei-Baffour, S. K. Amoah, C. Galbete, P. Henneman, K. Klipstein-Grobusch, M. Nicolaou, A. Adeyemo, J. van Straalen, L. Smeeth, and K. Stronks. 2016. Obesity and type 2 diabetes in sub-Saharan Africans—is the burden in today's Africa similar to African migrants in Europe? The RODAM study. *BMC Medicine* 14(1):166. doi: 10.1186/s12916-016-0709-0.

Anand, S. S., C. Hawkes, R. J. de Souza, A. Mente, M. Dehghan, R. Nugent, M. A. Zulyniak, T. Weis, A. M. Bernstein, R. M. Krauss, D. Kromhout, D. J. A. Jenkins, V. Malik, M. A. Martinez-Gonzalez, D. Mozaffarian, S. Yusuf, W. C. Willett, and B. M. Popkin. 2015. Food consumption and its impact on cardiovascular disease: Importance of solutions focused on the globalized food system: A report from the workshop convened by the World Heart Federation. *Journal of the American College of Cardiology* 66(14):1590–1614.

Anderson, I., B. Robson, M. Connolly, F. Al-Yaman, E. Bjertness, A. King, M. Tynan, R. Madden, A. Bang, C. E. Coimbra, Jr., M. A. Pesantes, H. Amigo, S. Andronov, B. Armien, D. A. Obando, P. Axelsson, Z. S. Bhatti, Z. A. Bhutta, P. Bjerregaard, M. B. Bjertness, R. Briceno-Leon, A. R. Broderstad, P. Bustos, V. Chongsuvivatwong, J. Chu, Deji, J. Gouda, R. Harikumar, T. T. Htay, A. S. Htet, C. Izugbara, M. Kamaka, M. King, M. R. Kodavanti, M. Lara, A. Laxmaiah, C. Lema, A. M. Taborda, T. Liabsuetrakul, A.

Lobanov, M. Melhus, I. Meshram, J. J. Miranda, T. T. Mu, B. Nagalla, A. Nimmathota, A. I. Popov, A. M. Poveda, F. Ram, H. Reich, R. V. Santos, A. A. Sein, C. Shekhar, L. Y. Sherpa, P. Skold, S. Tano, A. Tanywe, C. Ugwu, F. Ugwu, P. Vapattanawong, X. Wan, J. R. Welch, G. Yang, Z. Yang, and L. Yap. 2016. Indigenous and tribal peoples' health (the Lancet-Lowitja Institute global collaboration): A population study. *The Lancet* 388(10040):131–157.

Assmus, G., J. U. Farley, and D. R. Lehmann. 1984. How advertising affects sales: Meta-analysis of econometric results. *Journal of Marketing Research* 21(1):65–74.

Australian Bureau of Statistics. 2013. *Australian aboriginal and Torres Strait Islander health survey: First results, Australia, 2012–13. Overweight and obesity.* http://www.abs.gov.au/ausstats/abs@.nsf/Lookup/A07BD8674C37D838CA257C2F001459FA?opendocument (accessed January 3, 2019).

Barnes, P. M., P. F. Adams, and E. Powell-Griner. 2008. *Health characteristics of the Asian adult population: United States, 2004–2006.* Washington, DC: U.S. Department of Health and Human Services, Centers for Disease Control and Prevention.

Barquera, S., and M. White. 2018. Treating obesity seriously in Mexico: Realizing, much too late, action must be immediate. *Obesity (Silver Spring)* 26(10):1530–1531.

Barquera, S., K. Sánchez-Bazan, A. Carriedo, and B. Swinburn. 2018. The development of a national obesity and diabetes prevention and control strategy in Mexico: Actors, actions and conflicts of interest. Paper read at the UK Health Forum. Public health and the food and drinks industry: The governance and ethics of interaction. Lessons from research, policy and practice. Londres: UK Health Forum.

Burlingame, B., and S. Dernini. 2019. *Sustainable diets: Linking nutrition and food systems.* Boston, MA: CAB International.

CDC (Centers for Disease Control and Prevention). 2010. *Health characteristics of the American Indian and Alaska native adult population: United States, 2004–2008.* Table 4. https://minorityhealth.hhs.gov/omh/browse.aspx?lvl=4&lvlID=33 (accessed January 3, 2019).

CDC. 2016. *U.S. National Health Interview Survey, age-adjusted data for adults ages 18 y and over.* https://www.cdc.gov/nchs/nhis/shs/tables.htm (accessed January 3, 2019).

CDC. 2017a. *Adult obesity prevalence maps.* https://www.cdc.gov/obesity/data/prevalence-maps.html (accessed January 2, 2019).

CDC. 2017b. *Summary health statistics: National Health Interview Survey: 2015.* Table A-15. http://www.cdc.gov/nchs/nhis/shs/tables.htm (accessed January 3, 2019).

Cediel, G., M. Reyes, M. L. da Costa Louzada, E. Martinez Steele, C. A. Monteiro, C. Corvalan, and R. Uauy. 2018. Ultra-processed foods and added sugars in the Chilean diet (2010). *Public Health Nutrition* 21(1):125–133.

Colchero, M. A., B. M. Popkin, J. A. Rivera, and S. W. Ng. 2016. Beverage purchases from stores in Mexico under the excise tax on sugar sweetened beverages: Observational study. *British Medical Journal* 352:h6704.

Colchero, M. A., J. Rivera-Dommarco, B. M. Popkin, and S. W. Ng. 2017. In Mexico, evidence of sustained consumer response two years after implementing a sugar-sweetened beverage tax. *Health Affairs (Millwood)* 36(3):564–571.

Cornwell, B., E. Villamor, M. Mora-Plazas, C. Marin, C. A. Monteiro, and A. Baylin. 2018. Processed and ultra-processed foods are associated with lower-quality nutrient profiles in children from Colombia. *Public Health Nutrition* 21(1):142–147.

Costa Louzada. M. L., A. P. Martins, D. S. Canella, L. G. Baraldi, R. B. Levy, R. M. Claro, J. C. Moubarac, G. Cannon, and C. A. Monteiro. 2015. Ultra-processed foods and the nutritional dietary profile in Brazil. *Revista de Saude Publica* 49(38).

Cradock, A. L., P. J. Troped, B. Fields, S. J. Melly, S. V. Simms, F. Gimmler, and M. Fowler. 2009. Factors associated with federal transportation funding for local pedestrian and bicycle programming and facilities. *Journal of Public Health Policy* 30 (Suppl. 1):S38–S72.

Davis, B., and C. Carpenter. 2009. Proximity of fast-food restaurants to schools and adolescent obesity. *American Journal of Public Health* 99(3):505–510. doi: 10.2105/AJPH.2008.137638.

Deurenberg-Yap, M., G. Schmidt, W. A. van Staveren, and P. Deurenberg. 2000. The paradox of low body mass index and high body fat percentage among Chinese, Malays and Indians in Singapore. *International Journal of Obesity and Related Metabolic Disorders: Journal of the International Association for the Study of Obesity* 24(8):1011–1017.

ECLAC (Economic Commission for Latin America and the Caribbean). 2016. *The cost of the double burden of malnutrition: Social and economic impact.* Santiago, Chile: Economic Commission for Latin America and the Caribbean.

Euromonitor. 2018. *Market sizes- historical- total volume- kilograms or litres per capita- packaged food, soft drinks, and hot drinks.* London, UK: Euromonitor Passport International.

FAO (Food and Agriculture Organization), IFAD (International Fund for Agricultural Development), UNICEF (United Nations Children's Fund), WFP (World Food Programme), and WHO (World Health Organization). 2018. *The state of food security and nutrition in the world 2018. Building climate resilience for food security and nutrition.* http://www.fao.org/3/I9553EN/i9553en.pdf (accessed February 25, 2019).

Fardet, A. 2016. Minimally processed foods are more satiating and less hyperglycemic than ultra-processed foods: A preliminary study with 98 ready-to-eat foods. *Food & Function* 7(5):2338–2346.

Fardet, A., C. Mejean, H. Laboure, V. A. Andreeva, and G. Feron. 2017. The degree of processing of foods which are most widely consumed by the French elderly population is associated with satiety and glycemic potentials and nutrient profiles. *Food & Function* 8(2):651–658.

Fardet, A., S. Lakhssassi, and A. Briffaz. 2018. Beyond nutrient-based food indices: A data mining approach to search for a quantitative holistic index reflecting the degree of food processing and including physicochemical properties. *Food & Function* 9(1):561–572.

GBD (Global Burden of Disease) 2013 Mortality and Causes of Death Collaborators. 2015. Global, regional, and national age-sex specific all-cause and cause-specific mortality for 240 causes of death, 1990–2013: A systematic analysis for the Global Burden of Disease Study 2013. *The Lancet* 385(9963):117–171.

GBD 2016 Risk Factors Collaborators. 2017. Global, regional, and national comparative risk assessment of 84 behavioural, environmental and occupational, and metabolic risks or clusters of risks, 1990–2016: A systematic analysis for the Global Burden of Disease Study 2016. *The Lancet* 390(10100):1345–1422.

Giles-Corti, B., J. Kerr, and M. Pratt. 2017. Supplement: Promoting physical activity in public spaces to advance a culture of health. *Preventive Medicine* 103:S1–S104.

Gombi-Vaca, M. F., R. Sichieri, and E. Verly, Jr. 2016. Caloric compensation for sugar-sweetened beverages in meals: A population-based study in Brazil. *Appetite* 98:67–73. doi: 10.1016/j.appet.2015.12.014.

Goryakin, Y., and M. Suhrcke. 2014. Economic development, urbanization, technological change and overweight: What do we learn from 244 demographic and health surveys? *Economics and Human Biology* 14:109–127. doi: 10.1016/j.ehb.2013.11.003.

Guerrero-Lopez, C. M., M. Molina, and M. A. Colchero. 2017. Employment changes associated with the introduction of taxes on sugar-sweetened beverages and nonessential energy-dense food in Mexico. *Preventive Medicine* 105S:S43–S49.

Gujral, U. P., E. Vittinghoff, M. Mongraw-Chaffin, D. Vaidya, N. R. Kandula, M. Allison, J. Carr, K. Liu, K. M. V. Narayan, and A. M. Kanaya. 2017. Cardiometabolic abnormalities among normal-weight persons from five racial/ethnic groups in the United States: A cross-sectional analysis of two cohort studies. *Annals of Internal Medicine* 166(9):628–636.

Gujral, U. P., V. Mohan, R. Pradeepa, M. Deepa, R. M. Anjana, and K. M. Narayan. 2018. Ethnic differences in the prevalence of diabetes in underweight and normal weight individuals: The CARRS and NHANES studies. *Diabetes Research and Clinical Practice* 146:34–40. doi: 10.1016/j.diabres.2018.09.011.

Guthold, R., G. A. Stevens, L. M. Riley, and F. C. Bull. 2018. Worldwide trends in insufficient physical activity from 2001 to 2016: A pooled analysis of 358 population-based surveys with 1.9 million participants. *Lancet Global Health* 6(10):e1077–e1086.

Hales, C. M., M. D. Carroll, C. D. Fryar, and C. L. Ogden. 2017. *Prevalence of obesity among adults and youth: United States, 2015–2016.* Washington, DC: U.S. Department of Health and Human Services, Centers for Disease Control and Prevention.

HHS (U.S. Department of Health and Human Services). 1996. *Physical activity and health: A report of the surgeon general.* Atlanta, GA: U.S. Department of Health and Human Services, Centers for Disease Control and Prevention, National Center for Chronic Disease Prevention and Health Promotion.

Hoyer, W. D. 1984. An examination of consumer decision making for a common repeat purchase product. *Journal of Consumer Research* 11(3):822–829.

IDF (International Diabetes Federation). 2017. *International diabetes atlas.* http://www.diabetesatlas.org/across-the-globe.html (accessed January 2, 2019).

IDF. 2018. *Facts and figures.* https://idf.org/52-about-diabetes.html (accessed January 2, 2019).

IHME (Institute for Health Metrics and Evaluation). 2018. *Global burden of disease (GBD) compare | viz hub.* https://vizhub.healthdata.org/gbd-compare (accessed January 2, 2018).

Jaacks, L. M., M. M. Slining, and B. M. Popkin. 2015. Recent underweight and overweight trends by rural-urban residence among women in low- and middle-income countries. *The Journal of Nutrition* 145(2):352–357.

Julia, C., L. Martinez, B. Alles, M. Touvier, S. Hercberg, C. Mejean, and E. Kesse-Guyot. 2018. Contribution of ultra-processed foods in the diet of adults from the French NutriNet-Santé study. *Public Health Nutrition* 21(1):27–37.

Juul, F., and E. Hemmingsson. 2015. Trends in consumption of ultra-processed foods and obesity in Sweden between 1960 and 2010. *Public Health Nutrition* 18(17):3096–3107.

Kandala, N. B., and S. Stranges. 2014. Geographic variation of overweight and obesity among women in Nigeria: A case for nutritional transition in sub-Saharan Africa. *PLoS One* 9(6):e101103.

Kelly, B., J. C. Halford, E. J. Boyland, K. Chapman, I. Bautista-Castano, C. Berg, M. Caroli, B. Cook, J. G. Coutinho, T. Effertz, E. Grammatikaki, K. Keller, R. Leung, Y. Manios, R. Monteiro, C. Pedley, H. Prell, K. Raine, E. Recine, L. Serra-Majem, S. Singh, and C. Summerbell. 2010. Television food advertising to children: A global perspective. *American Journal of Public Health* 100(9):1730–1736.

Keybridge. 2018. *2025 beverage calories initiative: Report on 2017 progress toward the community calorie goal.* https://www.healthiergeneration.org/sites/default/files/documents/20181127/34111daa/BCI%202017%20Community%20Progress%20Report_AHG.pdf (accessed December 12, 2018).

Kuhnlein, H. V., B. Erasmus, and D. Spigelski. 2009. *Indigenous peoples' food systems: The many dimensions of culture, diversity and environment for nutrition and health.* Rome, Italy: Food and Agriculture Organization of the United Nations.

Kuhnlein, H. V., B. Erasmus, D. Spigelski, and B. Burlingame. 2013. *Indigenous peoples: Food systems and well-being: Interventions and policies for healthy communities.* Rome, Italy: Food and Agriculture Organization of the United Nations.

Kumanyika, S. 2018. K–9 unraveling common threads in obesity risk among racial/ethnic minority and migrant populations. *European Journal of Public Health* 28(Suppl. 1):cky044.009. doi: 10.1093/eurpub/cky044.009.

Kumanyika, S., W. C. Taylor, S. A. Grier, V. Lassiter, K. J. Lancaster, C. B. Morssink, and A. M. Renzaho. 2012. Community energy balance: A framework for contextualizing cultural influences on high risk of obesity in ethnic minority populations. *Preventive Medicine* 55(5):371–381.

Lakshmi, S., B. Metcalf, C. Joglekar, C. S. Yajnik, C. H. Fall, and T. J. Wilkin. 2012. Differences in body composition and metabolic status between white U.K. and Asian Indian children (EarlyBird 24 and the Pune Maternal Nutrition Study). *Pediatric Obesity* 7(5):347–354.

Lapierre, M. A., S. E. Vaala, and D. L. Linebarger. 2011. Influence of licensed spokescharacters and health cues on children's ratings of cereal taste. *Archives of Pediatric and Adolescent Medicine* 165(3):229–234. doi: 10.1001/archpediatrics.2010.300.

Lemke, S., and T. Delormier. 2017. Indigenous peoples' food systems, nutrition, and gender: Conceptual and methodological considerations. *Maternal & Child Nutrition* 13(Suppl. 3). doi: 10.1111/mcn.12499.

Locke, A. E., B. Kahali, S. I. Berndt, A. E. Justice, T. H. Pers, F. R. Day, C. Powell, S. Vedantam, M. L. Buchkovich, J. Yang, et al. 2015. Genetic studies of body mass index yield new insights for obesity biology. *Nature* 518(7538):197–206.

Loring, B., and A. Robertson. 2014. *Obesity and inequities. Guidance for addressing inequities in overweight and obesity.* Copenhagen, Denmark: World Health Organization Regional Office for Europe.

Mandrioli, D., C. E. Kearns, and L. A. Bero. 2016. Relationship between research outcomes and risk of bias, study sponsorship, and author financial conflicts of interest in reviews of the effects of artificially sweetened beverages on weight outcomes: A systematic review of reviews. *PLoS One* 11(9):e0162198.

Martinez Steele, E., L. G. Baraldi, M. L. Louzada, J. C. Moubarac, D. Mozaffarian, and C. A. Monteiro. 2016. Ultra-processed foods and added sugars in the U.S. diet: Evidence from a nationally representative cross-sectional study. *BMJ Open* 6(3):e009892.

Meeks, K. A. C., P. Henneman, A. Venema, T. Burr, C. Galbete, I. Danquah, M. B. Schulze, F. P. Mockenhaupt, E. Owusu-Dabo, C. N. Rotimi, J. Addo, L. Smeeth, S. Bahendeka, J. Spranger, M. Mannens, M. H. Zafarmand, C. Agyemang, and A. Adeyemo. 2017. An epigenome-wide association study in whole blood of measures of adiposity among Ghanaians: The RODAM study. *Clinical Epigenetics* 9:103. doi: 10.1186/s13148-017-0403-x.

Ministry of Health of Brazil. 2015. *Dietary guidelines for the Brazilian population.* Brazil: Ministry of Health of Brazil.

Monteiro, C. A., J. C. Moubarac, R. B. Levy, D. S. Canella, M. Louzada, and G. Cannon. 2018. Household availability of ultra-processed foods and obesity in nineteen European countries. *Public Health Nutrition* 21(1):18–26.

National Center for Chronic and Noncommunicable Disease Control and Prevention. 2016. *Report on the chronic disease risk factor surveillance in China 2013.* Beijing, China: National Center for Chronic Noncommunicable Diseases Control and Prevention.

NCD-RisC (Noncommunicable Disease Risk Factor Collaboration). 2016. Trends in adult body-mass index in 200 countries from 1975 to 2014: A pooled analysis of 1698 population-based measurement studies with 19.2 million participants. *The Lancet* 387(10026):1377–1396.

NCD-RisC. 2017. Worldwide trends in body-mass index, underweight, overweight, and obesity from 1975 to 2016: A pooled analysis of 2416 population-based measurement studies in 128.9 million children, adolescents, and adults. *The Lancet* 390(10113):2627–2642.

New Zealand Ministry of Health. 2018. *New Zealand health survey, 2016–2017; age-adjusted data for adults ages 15+y*. https://minhealthnz.shinyapps.io/nz-health-survey-2016-17-annual-data-explorer/_w_e5196d0b/_w_6cb88ed7/_w_4799831a/#!/explore-indicators (accessed January 3, 2019).

Nyberg, S. T., G. D. Batty, J. Pentti, M. Virtanen, L. Alfredsson, E. I. Fransson, M. Goldberg, K. Heikkila, M. Jokela, A. Knutsson, M. Koskenvuo, T. Lallukka, C. Leineweber, J. V. Lindbohm, I. E. H. Madsen, L. L. Magnusson Hanson, M. Nordin, T. Oksanen, O. Pietilainen, O. Rahkonen, R. Rugulies, M. J. Shipley, S. Stenholm, S. Suominen, T. Theorell, J. Vahtera, P. J. M. Westerholm, H. Westerlund, M. Zins, M. Hamer, A. Singh-Manoux, J. A. Bell, J. E. Ferrie, and M. Kivimaki. 2018. Obesity and loss of disease-free years owing to major non-communicable diseases: A multicohort study. *The Lancet Public Health* 3(10):e490–e497.

OECD (Organisation for Economic Co-operation and Development). 2017. *OECD health statistics 2017*. https://dx.doi.org/10.1787/888933602956 (accessed January 3, 2019).

PAHO (Pan American Health Organization). 2015. *Ultra-processed food and drink products in Latin America: Trends, impact on obesity, policy implications*. Washington, DC: Pan American Health Organization.

Patel, S. A., K. M. Narayan, and S. A. Cunningham. 2015. Unhealthy weight among children and adults in India: Urbanicity and the crossover in underweight and overweight. *Annals of Epidemiology*. 25(5):336–341.e332. doi: 10.1016/j.annepidem.2015.02.009.

Paul, P., S. A. Carlson, D. D. Carroll, D. Berrigan, and J. E. Fulton. 2015. Walking for transportation and leisure among U.S. adults—National Health Interview Survey 2010. *Journal of Physical Activity and Health* 12:S62–S69.

Popejoy, A. B., and S. M. Fullerton. 2016. Genomics is failing on diversity. *Nature* 538(7624):161–164.

Popkin, B. M., S. Horton, S. Kim, A. Mahal, and J. Shuigao. 2001. Trends in diet, nutritional status, and diet-related noncommunicable diseases in China and India: The economic costs of the nutrition transition. *Nutrition Reviews* 59(12):379–390.

Popkin, B. M., S. Kim, E. R. Rusev, S. Du, and C. Zizza. 2006. Measuring the full economic costs of diet, physical activity and obesity-related chronic diseases. *Obesity Reviews* 7(3):271–293.

Public Health England. 2016. *Adult obesity slide set*. http://webarchive.nationalarchives.gov.uk/20170110165555/https://www.noo.org.uk/slide_sets (accessed January 3, 2019).

Public Health England. 2018. *Sugar reduction and wider reformulation programme: Report on progress towards the first 5% reduction and next steps*. London, UK: Public Health England.

Pucher, J., J. Dill, and S. Handy. 2010. Infrastructure, programs, and policies to increase bicycling: An international review. *Preventive Medicine* 50:S106–S125.

Rachele, J. N., T. Sugiyama, G. Turrell, A. M. Healy, and J. F. Sallis. 2018. Automobile dependence: A contributing factor to poorer health among lower-income households. *Journal of Transport and Health* 8:123–128.

Razak, F., S. S. Anand, H. Shannon, V. Vuksan, B. Davis, R. Jacobs, K. K. Teo, M. McQueen, and S. Yusuf. 2007. Defining obesity cut points in a multiethnic population. *Circulation* 115(16):2111–2118.

Ritchie, H., and M. Roser. 2018. *Obesity*. https://ourworldindata.org/obesity#data-sources (accessed January 2, 2019).

Ruel, M. T., and H. Alderman. 2013. Nutrition-sensitive interventions and programmes: How can they help to accelerate progress in improving maternal and child nutrition? *The Lancet* 382(9891):536–551.

Sattar, N., and J. M. Gill. 2015. Type 2 diabetes in migrant south Asians: Mechanisms, mitigation, and management. *The Lancet. Diabetes & Endocrinology* 3(12):1004–1016.

REFERENCES

Schmengler, H., U. Z. Ikram, M. B. Snijder, A. E. Kunst, and C. Agyemang. 2017. Association of perceived ethnic discrimination with general and abdominal obesity in ethnic minority groups: The HELIUS study. *Journal of Epidemiology and Community Health* 71(5):453–460.

Serodio, P. M., M. McKee, and D. Stuckler. 2018. Coca-Cola—a model of transparency in research partnerships? A network analysis of Coca-Cola's research funding (2008–2016). *Public Health Nutrition* 21(9):1594–1607.

Shekar, M., J. Kakietek, J. Dayton Eberwein, and D. Walters. 2017. *An investment framework for nutrition: Reaching the global targets for stunting, anemia, breastfeeding, and wasting*. http://www.worldbank.org/en/topic/nutrition/publication/an-investment-framework-for-nutrition-reaching-the-global-targets-for-stunting-anemia-breastfeeding-wasting (accessed February 25, 2019).

Silver, L. D., S. W. Ng, S. Ryan-Ibarra, L. S. Taillie, M. Induni, D. R. Miles, J. M. Poti, and B. M. Popkin. 2017. Changes in prices, sales, consumer spending, and beverage consumption one year after a tax on sugar-sweetened beverages in Berkeley, California, U.S.: A before-and-after study. *PLoS Medicine* 14(4):e1002283.

Simon, P. 2012. Collecting ethnic statistics in Europe: A review. *Ethnic and Racial Studies* 35(8):1366–1391.

Snijder, M. B., H. Galenkamp, M. Prins, E. M. Derks, R. J. G. Peters, A. H. Zwinderman, and K. Stronks. 2017. Cohort profile: The healthy life in an urban setting (HELIUS) study in Amsterdam, the Netherlands. *BMJ Open* 7(12):e017873.

Solar, O., and A. Irwin. 2010. *A conceptual framework for action on the social determinants of health*. Geneva, Switzerland: World Health Organization. https://www.who.int/sdhconference/resources/ConceptualframeworkforactiononSDH_eng.pdf (accessed February 27, 2019).

Stern, D., L. Tolentino, and S. Barquera. 2011. *Front labeling review: Analysis of the daily dietary guidelines and their understanding by nutrition students in Mexico*. Mexico: Instituto Nacional de Salud Pública.

Thomasson, E. 2012. Insight—at Nestle, interacting with the online enemy. *Reuters*, October 26. https://uk.reuters.com/article/uk-nestle-online-water/insight-at-nestle-interacting-with-the-online-enemy-idUKBRE89P07Q20121026 (accessed January 9, 2019).

UN (United Nations). 2009. *State of the world's Indigenous Peoples*. Vol. 1. New York: United Nations. https://www.un.org/esa/socdev/unpfii/documents/SOWIP/en/SOWIP_web.pdf (accessed February 27, 2019).

UN. 2013. *State of the world's Indigenous Peoples: Indigenous Peoples' access to health services*. New York: United Nations. https://www.un.org/development/desa/indigenous-peoples/wp-content/uploads/sites/19/2018/03/The-State-of-The-Worlds-Indigenous-Peoples-WEB.pdf (accessed February 27, 2019).

UN. 2017a. *International migration report*. New York: United Nations. http://www.un.org/en/development/desa/population/migration/publications/migrationreport/docs/MigrationReport2017_Highlights.pdf (accessed February 27, 2019).

UN. 2017b. *State of the world's indigenous peoples: Education*, Vol. 3. ST/ESA/368. New York: United Nations. https://www.un.org/development/desa/indigenouspeoples/wp-content/uploads/sites/19/2017/12/State-of-Worlds-Indigenous-Peoples_III_WEB2018.pdf (accessed February 27, 2019).

WCRFI (World Cancer Research Fund International). 2018. NOURISHING database. https://www.wcrf.org/int/policy/nourishing-database (accessed January 3, 2019).

WHO (World Health Organization). 2004. *Global strategy on diet, physical activity, and health*. Geneva, Switzerland: World Health Organization.

WHO. 2011. *Waist circumference and waist-hip ratio: Report of a WHO expert consultation, Geneva, 8–11 December 2008.* https://apps.who.int/iris/bitstream/handle/10665/44583/9789241501491_eng.pdf;jsessionid=AF20412B758FD03581101EDB45E83485?sequence=1 (accessed February 25, 2019).
WHO. 2013. *Global action plan for the prevention and control of NCDs 2013–2020.* Geneva, Switzerland: World Health Organization.
WHO. 2016a. *Global report on diabetes.* Geneva, Switzerland: World Health Organization.
WHO. 2016b. *Report of the commission on ending childhood obesity.* Geneva, Switzerland: World Health Organization.
WHO. 2017. *Double-duty actions for nutrition: Policy brief.* Geneva, Switzerland: World Health Organization.
WHO. 2018a. *Global action plan on physical activity 2018–2030: More active people for a healthier world.* Geneva, Switzerland: World Health Organization.
WHO. 2018b. *Obesity and overweight.* https://www.who.int/en/news-room/fact-sheets/detail/obesity-and-overweight (accessed January 7, 2019).
WHO Expert Consultation. 2004. Appropriate body-mass index for Asian populations and its implications for policy and intervention strategies. *The Lancet* 363(9403):157–163.
Woodside, A. G., and G. I. Waddle. 1975. Sales effects of in-store advertising. *Journal of Advertising Research* 15(3):29–33.
Yoon, K. H., J. H. Lee, J. W. Kim, J. H. Cho, Y. H. Choi, S. H. Ko, P. Zimmet, and H. Y. Son. 2006. Epidemic obesity and type 2 diabetes in Asia. *The Lancet* 368(9548):1681–1688.

A

Workshop Agenda

Current Status and Response to the Global Obesity Pandemic:
A Workshop

Roundtable on Obesity Solutions

October 9, 2018

National Academy of Sciences Building
2101 Constitution Avenue, NW, Washington, DC
Lecture Room

8:30 AM	Welcome
	Bill Purcell, Chair, Roundtable on Obesity Solutions

SESSION 1: State of Obesity Globally

8:40 AM	Moderator: *Christina Economos, Tufts University*

Lindsay Jaacks, Harvard T.H. Chan School of Public Health
Vasanti Malik, Harvard T.H. Chan School of Public Health
Karlijn Meeks, Academic Medical Center, Netherlands
Rachel Nugent, RTI International

Session Discussion

10:25 AM	BREAK

SESSION 2: Global Obesity Prevention and Treatment Efforts

10:40 AM	Moderator: *James Sallis, University of California, San Diego*

> Olivia Barata Cavalcanti, World Obesity Federation
> Fiona Bull, World Health Organization (videoconference)
> Fabio da Silva Gomes, Pan American Health
>   Organization/World Health Organization
>
> Session Discussion

12:00 PM   LUNCH

SESSION 3: Challenges

1:00 PM   Moderator: *Rachel Nugent, RTI International*

> **Navigating the Obesity Epidemic: The Mexico Experience**
> *Simón Barquera, Mexican National Institute of Public Health*
>
> **Cross-Cultural Insights About Obesity Research, Policy, and Practice Related to High-Risk Populations**
> *Shiriki Kumanyika, Drexel University*
> *Harriet Kuhnlein, Emeritus, McGill University*
>
> Session Discussion

2:30 PM   BREAK

SESSION 4: Next Steps

2:45 PM   Moderator: *Bill Dietz, The George Washington University*

> *James Sallis, University of California, San Diego*
> *Neena Prasad, Bloomberg Philanthropies*
> *Meera Shekar, World Bank*
> *Bill Dietz, The George Washington University*
>
> Session Discussion

4:00 PM   Workshop Adjourns

B

Acronyms and Abbreviations

BMI	body mass index
CDC	U.S. Centers for Disease Control and Prevention
ECLAC	Economic Commission for Latin America and the Caribbean
FAO	Food and Agriculture Organization
GDA	Guideline Daily Amount
GDP	gross domestic product
HELIUS	Healthy Life in an Urban Setting
IDF	International Diabetes Federation
IHME	Institute for Health Metrics and Evaluation
MAPPS	Management Advocacy for Providers, Patients, and Systems
NCD	noncommunicable disease
NCD-RisC	Noncommunicable Diseases Risk Factor Collaboration
OECD	Organisation for Economic Co-operation and Development

PAHO	Pan American Health Organization
RODAM	Research on Obesity and Diabetes among African Migrants
UN	United Nations
WHO	World Health Organization
WHO-CHOICE	World Health Organization's CHOosing Interventions that are Cost-Effective

C

Biographical Sketches of Workshop Speakers and Planning Committee Members

Olivia Barata Cavalcanti, Dr.P.H., M.P.H., M.I.A., has almost a decade of experience in public health, with a special focus on obesity and public–private partnerships to fight noncommunicable diseases. As director of health systems and professional education for the World Obesity Federation, she leads the organization's training and certification program in obesity care, and is responsible for monitoring obesity prevention and treatment in health systems across the globe and strengthening policy and guidelines. She has worked for different international and nonprofit organizations in Italy, the United States, and the United Kingdom, where she was in charge of all aspects of the design and implementation of health programs on diabetes, obesity, and cardiovascular disease for both low-income children and adults. Dr. Barata Cavalcanti also has deep knowledge of and experience with the United Nations system, having worked at the Joint United Nations Programme on HIV/AIDS in Mozambique, for the U.S. Fund for United Nations Children's Fund, and as a fellow at the Italian Mission to the United Nations. She has experience teaching public health, community health, and research methods courses in various universities at both the undergraduate and graduate levels (Brooklyn College, Hunter College, and the City University of New York [CUNY] Graduate School of Public Health and Health Policy). She earned her doctorate of public health (Dr.P.H.) from CUNY Graduate School of Public Health and Health Policy. She also holds master of public health and master of international affairs degrees from Columbia University.

Simón Barquera, M.D., Ph.D., M.S., is director of the Nutrition and Health Research Center at Mexico's National Institute of Public Health, where he also leads the Obesity, Diabetes and Cardiovascular Disease research line. He has been a consultant for the World Health Organization, the Pan American Health Organization (PAHO), the United Nations Children's Fund, and the International Atomic Energy Agency in the fields of nutrition, obesity, and chronic diseases. He has published more than 251 research papers and chapters, and has more than 9,000 citations to his work. He is associate editor of *Public Health Nutrition* and editorial board member of *Global Health Epidemiology and Genomics*. Dr. Barquera is co-researcher of the Mexican Health and Nutrition Surveys (1999–2016); member of the Ministry of Health Chronic Diseases advisory board, the PAHO Expert Group on sodium reduction, and the World Obesity Federation Scientific Advisory Board; and fellow of the Obesity Society. He has been recognized as a top-level national researcher by Mexico's National Council of Science and Technology, and a fellow of the Mexican National Academy of Medicine and the Mexican Academy of Sciences. Among many other distinctions, he has received the PAHO Fred L. Soper Award for Excellence in Health Literature (2003), the Tufts University Nutrition Impact Award (2016), the Universidad Autónoma Metropolitana (UAM) Distinguished Alumni Award (2016), and the 11th Michael and Susan Dell Lectureship Award in Child Health (2017). He received his M.D. from UAM, Mexico City, and holds an M.S. and a Ph.D. in nutrition epidemiology from the Friedman School of Nutrition Science and Policy at Tufts University.

Fiona Bull, M.B.E., Ph.D., M.Sc., is programme manager in the Department of Prevention of Noncommunicable Diseases (NCDs) at the World Health Organization (WHO), based in Geneva, Switzerland. She leads WHO's global work on physical inactivity, healthy eating, and prevention of obesity, in addition to providing leadership for global monitoring and surveillance of NCDs and their risk factors. Dr. Bull joined WHO in January 2017 after 25 years in applied research in Australia, the United Kingdom, and the United States. Her recent positions include professor of public health and director of the Centre for Built Environment and Health at the University of Western Australia and professor of sports science and director of the National Centre of Physical Activity at Loughborough University in the United Kingdom. Throughout her career, Dr. Bull has focused on developing scientific evidence and understanding on healthy lifestyles to inform public policy and implementation of practical programs in community settings. Her work is multidisciplinary and includes contributions in the areas of the global burden of disease, national initiatives in worksites, primary health care, the built and natural environments, national surveillance initiatives, and policy evaluations across many settings. Dr. Bull has co-authored more than 180 scientific publications and reports. Her interest is in bridging the knowledge–policy practice gap, and she has been actively involved in civil society and is immediate past president of the International Society of Physical Activity. In 2014, Dr. Bull was named a Member of the British Empire (MBE) for her services to public health.

Fabio da Silva Gomes, Ph.D., has worked as a Ministry of Health senior officer in Brazil for 10 years, developing strategies for promoting healthy eating practices in multiple settings; mobilizing regulatory measures to reduce the demand for unhealthy products; and protecting health, food, and nutrition public policies from the interference of opposing commercial actors. He served on the Working Group on Implementation, Monitoring and Accountability of the Commission on Ending Childhood Obesity of the World Health Organization, and has advised and supported United Nations agencies; governments; social movements; and professional, scientific, and civil society organizations worldwide, including the World Public Health Nutrition Association and the World Obesity Federation. Dr. Gomes is now regional advisor on nutrition and physical activity for the Americas at the Pan American Health Organization/World Health Organization, supporting countries in designing and implementing food and nutrition public policies as well as protecting such policies from opposing interests. He is a nutritionist (Rio de Janeiro State University) with a master's degree in population studies and social research from the National School of Statistical Sciences of Brazil and a Ph.D. in public health from the Institute of Social Medicine of the Rio de Janeiro State University.

Bill Dietz, M.D., Ph.D., is a consultant to the Roundtable on Obesity Solutions of the National Academies of Sciences, Engineering, and Medicine and chair of the Sumner M. Redstone Global Center for Prevention and Wellness at the Milken Institute School of Public Health at The George Washington University. He was director of the Division of Nutrition, Physical Activity, and Obesity in the Center for Chronic Disease Prevention and Health Promotion at the Centers for Disease Control and Prevention (CDC) from 1997 to 2012. Prior to his appointment to CDC, he was a professor of pediatrics at the Tufts University School of Medicine and director of clinical nutrition at the Floating Hospital of New England Medical Center Hospitals. Dr. Dietz has been a counselor and is past president of the American Society for Clinical Nutrition, and is also past president of the North American Association for the Study of Obesity. From 2001 to 2003, he served as a member of the Advisory Board to the Institute of Nutrition, Metabolism, and Diabetes of the Canadian Institutes for Health Research. In 2000, Dr. Dietz received the William G. Anderson Award from the American Alliance for Health, Physical Education, Recreation and Dance, and was recognized for excellence in his work and advocacy by the Association of State and Territorial Public Health Nutrition Directors. In 2002, he was made an honorary member of the American Dietetic Association, and received the Holroyd-Sherry award for his outstanding contributions to the field of children, adolescents, and the media. In 2005 Dr. Dietz received the George Bray Founders Award from the North American Association for the Study of Obesity. In 2006 he received the Nutrition Award from the American Academy of Pediatrics for outstanding research related to nutrition of infants and children. In 2008 Dr. Dietz received the Oded Bar-Or award from the Obesity Society for excellence in pediatric obesity research. In 2012 he received a Special Recognition Award from the American Academy of Pediatrics Provisional Section on Obesity and the Outstanding Achievement Award from the Georgia Chapter of the American Academy of Pediatrics. Dr. Dietz is the author of more than 200 publications in the scientific literature and the editor of 5 books, including *Clinical Obesity in Adults and Children* and *Nutrition: What Every Parent Needs to Know*. He received his B.A. from Wesleyan University in 1966 and his M.D. from the University of Pennsylvania in 1970. After completing his residency at Upstate Medical Center, he received a Ph.D. in nutritional biochemistry from the Massachusetts Institute of Technology. Dr. Dietz is a member of the National Academy of Medicine.

Christina Economos, Ph.D., is co-founder and director of ChildObesity180 and is professor and New Balance chair in childhood nutrition at the Friedman School of Nutrition Science and Policy at Tufts University. As the principal investigator for large-scale research studies, Dr. Economos's goal is to inspire behavior, policy, and environmental change to reduce obesity and improve the health of America's children. At ChildObesity180, she blends scientific evidence and rigor with innovation and experience from the private sector to develop, implement, evaluate, and scale high-impact obesity prevention initiatives. She led the groundbreaking Shape Up Somerville study, demonstrating that it is possible to reduce excess weight gain in children through multiple leverage points within an entire community. Dr. Economos is involved in national obesity and public health activities and has served on four Institute of Medicine (now Health and Medicine Division) committees, including the Committee on Accelerating Progress in Obesity Prevention and the Committee on an Evidence-Based Framework for Obesity Prevention Decision Making. In addition, she serves on the American Heart Association's Nutrition Council on Lifestyle and Cardiometabolic Health, and has authored more than 130 scientific publications. Dr. Economos received a B.S. degree from Boston University, an M.S. degree in applied physiology and nutrition from Columbia University, and a Ph.D. in nutritional biochemistry from Tufts University.

Lindsay Jaacks, Ph.D., is assistant professor in the Department of Global Health and Population at the Harvard T.H. Chan School of Public Health and visiting professor at the Public Health Foundation of India in Delhi. Prior to her appointment at the Harvard T.H. Chan School of Public Health, she completed a postdoctoral fellowship at the Emory Global Diabetes Research Center in Atlanta. The overarching vision of Dr. Jaacks's research program is to advance knowledge of the intersection between the food system and the health system with respect to cardiometabolic health, and to apply that knowledge in developing interventions to halt the increase in obesity and diabetes, particularly in low- and middle-income countries. Dr. Jaacks has served as a consultant to the UK Department for International Development on addressing overweight/obesity in low-income countries, and is currently serving as a consultant to RTI International on estimating the impact of food and nutrition policies on diabetes. She is a fellow for the Lancet Commission on Obesity.

Harriet Kuhnlein, Ph.D., L.L.D. (hon.), F.A.S.N., F.I.U.N.S., is emerita professor at McGill University, Montreal. Dr. Kuhnlein has held professorial appointments at the University of British Columbia, the University of Hawaii at Manoa, and McGill University. She taught and conducted research at McGill's School of Human Nutrition in the Faculty of Agricultural and Environmental Sciences, the Faculty of Medicine, and the McGill School of the Environment. She is founding director of the Centre for Indigenous Peoples' Nutrition and Environment, an internationally recognized center for interdisciplinary participatory research and education related to Indigenous Peoples' food systems. Having engaged with communities of Indigenous Peoples in many parts of the world for more than 40 years, she is recognized for unique pioneering expertise that has led to the identification, characterization, and preservation of traditional food systems of Indigenous Peoples throughout the world, and to growing recognition that these ecosystems are important for health and well-being. Her publications include nearly 400 journal articles, books, book chapters, abstracts, and conference proceedings. Notably, Dr. Kuhnlein has inspired a new generation of nutrition scientists who are champions of participatory research and Indigenous Peoples' nutrition and food security. She is a fellow of the American Society of Nutrition and honorary member of the Canadian Nutrition Society, fellow of the International Union of Nutritional Sciences (IUNS), and member of the IUNS Task Force on Traditional and Indigenous Food Systems and Nutrition. Recently, she was a 2017 Fulbright Global/Public Health Specialist Grant recipient at Massey University in Wellington, New Zealand. She is active with the Board of Trustees of the International Foundation for Science (Stockholm), the Lancet Commission on Obesity, and the Planning Committee of the Native American Nutrition Conferences

(United States). Dr. Kuhnlein has contributed to many consultancies and served on several national and international committees, especially those related to food data and nutrition of Indigenous Peoples. She holds a Ph.D. from the University of California, Berkeley, and an honorary doctor of laws degree from the University of Western Ontario.

Shiriki Kumanyika, Ph.D., M.P.H., M.S.W., is research professor in the Department of Community Health and Prevention at the Drexel Dornsife School of Public Health, Drexel University, and emeritus professor of epidemiology at the Perelman School of Medicine, University of Pennsylvania. Dr. Kumanyika has a unique interdisciplinary background that integrates epidemiology, nutrition, social work, and public health methods and perspectives. The main themes of her research concern prevention and control of obesity and other diet-related risk factors and chronic diseases, with a particular focus on reducing the prevalence and health burdens of obesity in black communities. In 2002, she formed the African American Collaborative Obesity Research Network (AACORN), a national network of academic scholars and community research partners who generate and translate research on nutrition, physical activity, and weight issues in African American children and adults. AACORN, now known as the Council on Black Health, has its national office at the Drexel Dornsife School. Dr. Kumanyika is a past president of the American Public Health Association and has served in numerous advisory roles related to public health research and policy in the United States and abroad. She is currently co-chair of the Policy and Prevention Section of the World Obesity Federation, a member of the Lancet Commission on Obesity, and a nutrition advisor to the World Health Organization. She has served on the Food and Nutrition Board and a number of National Academies of Sciences, Engineering, and Medicine study committees, such as the Committee for Prevention of Obesity in Children and Youth (member), the Committee on Progress in Preventing Childhood Obesity (volunteer consultant), the Committee on an Evidence-Based Framework for Obesity Prevention Decision Making (chair), and the Committee on Accelerating Progress in Obesity Prevention (member). Dr. Kumanyika also chaired the Standing Committee on Childhood Obesity Prevention from 2009 until its retirement in 2013. She received her M.S. in social work from Columbia University, an M.P.H. from Johns Hopkins University, and a Ph.D. in human nutrition from Cornell University. She is a member of the National Academy of Medicine.

Tim Lobstein, Ph.D., is a United Kingdom and United States dual national with policy expertise in the field of obesity and diet-related disease. He is policy director for the World Obesity Federation, based in London, and an occasional consultant to the World Health Organization, the European Commission (EC), the UK government's Public Health England, and various other international authorities and nongovernmental organizations. Dr. Lobstein is a visiting professor at the Public Health Advocacy Institute of Western Australia, Curtin University, and at the Boden Institute, University of Sydney, New South Wales. He is the author of chapters on food policy and obesity in international textbooks, the author or co-author of more than 30 papers in peer-reviewed journals, and the author of several popular books on food and nutrition. Dr. Lobstein has undertaken research projects funded by the EC on health inequalities and income disparities and on marketing of food and beverages to children, and has been a work-package leader on six EC-funded FP6, FP7, and H2020 projects related to nutrition, the prevention and management of obesity, and health impact assessment. He has extensive experience in policy analysis, policy dissemination, evidence reviews, and knowledge transfer.

Vasanti Malik, Sc.D., is a research scientist in the Department of Nutrition at the Harvard T.H. Chan School of Public Health. Her research focuses on evaluating risk factors for obesity, type 2 diabetes, and cardiovascular disease, with an emphasis on diet quality. Among her research areas, Dr. Malik is most known for her work related to sugary beverages, which has had an important role in shaping dietary recommendations and policies for reducing intake. She also studies nutritional drivers of the global obesity and diabetes epidemics in countries undergoing epidemiologic transition, and currently directs the Global Nutrition and Epidemiologic Transition Initiative, a collaborative project involving 13 low- and middle-income countries that aims to reduce diabetes risk by improving diet and lifestyle. She is an associate editor for *BMC Obesity* and a review editor for *Frontiers in Public Health*. The ultimate goal of Dr. Malik's work is to inform future large-scale community-based interventions and policy strategies for reducing the risk of obesity and related chronic diseases nationally and internationally. She obtained an M.Sc. in nutritional sciences from the University of Toronto and a dual doctorate in nutrition and epidemiology from the Harvard T.H. Chan School of Public Health.

Karlijn Meeks, Ph.D., M.Sc., is a postdoctoral research fellow at the Department of Public Health, Academic Medical Center-University of Amsterdam (AMC-UvA), the Netherlands. Her work focuses on the complex interplay between genetic and environmental factors contributing to noncommunicable diseases in African populations. Between 2013 and 2017, she was a Ph.D. candidate in the Department of Public Health, AMC-UvA. Her Ph.D. work was embedded within the multicenter Research on Obesity and Diabetes among African Migrants (RODAM) study. That study collected data among African migrants in three European countries, as well as among Africans in urban and rural Africa. In 2015, Dr. Meeks won the AMC Young Talent Fund Award, which provided her the opportunity to be trained in the field of (epi)genetics at the Center for Research on Genomics and Global Health, National Institutes of Health. In 2017 she successfully defended her Ph.D. thesis, entitled "Epidemiology and Epigenetics of Type 2 Diabetes among African Migrants in Europe." After completing her Ph.D., she obtained a grant to continue her work on African populations at AMC-UvA for 1 year as a postdoctoral research fellow. As part of this postdoctoral position, she spent some time as a visiting research fellow in the Global Health and Populations Department, Wellcome Trust Sanger Institute, United Kingdom. Dr. Meeks received her B.S. (2010) and M.S. (2012) in nutrition and health from Wageningen University, the Netherlands, and her Ph.D. from the University of Amsterdam.

Rachel Nugent, M.Phil., Ph.D., is vice president for global noncommunicable diseases (NCDs) at RTI International. She joined RTI in February 2016 to lead a global initiative to prevent and reduce the health and economic burdens of NCDs in low- and middle-income countries. Prior to this position, Dr. Nugent was associate professor in the Department of Global Health at the University of Washington and director of the Disease Control Priorities Network. She has advised the World Health Organization (WHO), the U.S. government, and nonprofit organizations on the economics and policy environment of NCDs. She is a member of WHO's Expert Advisory Panel on Management of NCDs, the Abraaj Health Care Fund Social Impact Committee, and the Lancet Commission on NCDIs of the Poorest Billion. She led a Lancet Task Force and Series on NCDs and Economics (2018). She served on the U.S. Institute of Medicine (IOM) (now Health and Medicine Division) Committee on Economic Evaluation for Investments in Children, Youth, and Families (2015–2016), was co-chair of the IOM Workshop on Country-Level Decision Making for Control of Chronic Diseases (2012), and was a member of the IOM Committee on Promoting Cardiovascular Health in the Developing World (2008–2010). Dr. Nugent focuses on using economic analysis for priority setting in health, and has worked with global and national institutions to increase the use of evidence for decision making. Her recent work includes tracking donor funding on NCDs, and assessing costs and benefits of NCD policies and interventions. She received her M.Phil. and Ph.D. degrees in economics from The George Washington University in Washington, DC.

Neena Prasad, M.D., M.P.H., M.Sc., joined the Public Health team of Bloomberg Philanthropies (BP) in 2008. She directs BP's Global Obesity Prevention and Maternal & Reproductive Health Programs. Dr. Prasad is also a key member of the Tobacco Control team, overseeing activities in India. Previously, she worked as a primary care physician serving inner-city populations at St. Michael's Hospital in Toronto and concurrently held the rank of assistant professor in the Department of Family and Community Medicine, University of Toronto. She holds an M.Sc. in psychiatry and behavioral neurosciences from McMaster University, an M.D. also from McMaster University, and an M.P.H. with a concentration in international health from the Harvard T.H. Chan School of Public Health.

Bill Purcell, J.D., is chair, Roundtable on Obesity Solutions at the National Academies of Sciences, Engineering, and Medicine; an attorney in Nashville, Tennessee; and an adjunct professor of public policy at Vanderbilt University. While he was serving as Mayor of Nashville (1999 to 2007), his accomplishments as a civic leader earned him Public Official of the Year honors in 2006 from *Governing Magazine*. Elected to five terms in the Tennessee House, he held the positions of majority leader and chair of the Select Committee on Children and Youth. After retiring from the General Assembly, Mr. Purcell founded and became director of the Child and Family Policy Center at the Vanderbilt Institute of Public Policy Studies. From 2008 to 2010, he served as director of the Institute of Politics at the Harvard Kennedy School of Government. He was then appointed special advisor and co-chair of the Work Team for Allston in the Office of the President at Harvard University. He previously served in various capacities on obesity-related committees of the National Academies, including the Committee on an Evidence-Based Framework for Obesity Prevention Decision Making (member), the Committee on Accelerating Progress in Obesity Prevention (vice chair), and the Standing Committee on Childhood Obesity Prevention (member). He graduated from Hamilton College and Vanderbilt University School of Law.

Nancy Roman, M.A., president and chief executive officer (CEO) of the Partnership for a Healthier America (PHA), joined the organization in September 2017 following an international career spanning journalism, business, and public service with the U.S. government and the United Nations. Prior to joining PHA, Ms. Roman was president and CEO of the Capital Area Food Bank (CAFB), the Washington, DC, region's largest organization working to solve hunger and its companion problems: chronic undernutrition and diet-related health issues such as heart disease and obesity. CAFB annually provides food and nutrition resources to 540,000 people—12 percent of the region's total population—through 444 partner nonprofits in the District, Northern Virginia, and Maryland. Under Ms. Roman's leadership, the food bank became a national voice for embedding health and wellness in hunger relief work. During her tenure, it dramatically increased the healthfulness of its food inventory by working with its corporate retail partners; pioneered new delivery models for fruits, vegetables, and nutrition resources; and advocated for access to affordable groceries in low-income areas through both existing and innovative models. Ms. Roman currently serves on the board of trustees of Global Communities, an international nongovernmental organization that works on hunger, health, microfinance, and lending to support lives and livelihoods, as well as on the board of trustees of the Millennial Action Project, which organizes nonpartisan communities to find common ground on the issues facing millennials and future generations. She holds an M.A. in international economics and American foreign policy from the Johns Hopkins School of Advanced International Studies and a B.A. in journalism and French from Baylor University.

James F. Sallis, Ph.D., is distinguished professor emeritus of family medicine and public health at the University of California, San Diego, and professorial fellow at the Australian Catholic University, Melbourne. His research interests are promoting physical activity and understanding policy and environmental influences on physical activity, nutrition, and obesity. He co-leads the International Physical Activity and Environment Network, which coordinates international studies with more than 20 countries. He has authored 700 scientific publications and is one of the world's most cited authors in the social sciences. Dr. Sallis is past president of the Society of Behavioral Medicine and a member of the National Academy of Medicine.

Meera Shekar, Ph.D., is global lead for nutrition with the World Bank's (the Bank's) Health, Nutrition and Population Global Practice. In this capacity she provides leadership, support, and policy advice on the Bank's nutrition portfolio across the spectrum of undernutrition and obesity, managing key partnerships such as the Power of Nutrition and the Japan Trust Fund, and firmly positioning nutrition within the Global Financing Facility for Reproductive, Maternal, Neonatal, Child, and Adolescent Health and the Bank's new initiative on human capital. She is also responsible for building cross-sectoral linkages with the agriculture, water and sanitation, education, and social protection Global Practices. During the past several years, she led a repositioning of the nutrition agenda that resulted in the establishment of the new global Scaling Up Nutrition (SUN) initiative and was a key partner in the discussions on the Catalytic Financing Facility for Nutrition, developed in partnership with the Milken Institute, which evolved into the Power of Nutrition. Dr. Shekar serves on the SUN executive committee and has been one of the principals for the emerging SUN aid-architecture and the G8 and G20 agenda-setting process for food security and nutrition over the past several years. She leads the global and country-level costing and financing analyses at the Bank and the first-ever global Investment Framework for Nutrition, and is leading the Bank's analytics on obesity prevention. She has also worked on the demographic dividend and population and development issues. Dr. Shekar has lived and worked across the globe and has extensive policy and operational experience in India, Bangladesh, Ethiopia, Nigeria, Tanzania, Vietnam, Bolivia, Guatemala, Uzbekistan, Sri Lanka, and the Philippines. Before joining the Bank in 2003, she led United Nations Children's Fund's Health, Nutrition, Water and Sanitation, and Early Childhood Development teams in Tanzania and the Philippines. Among other publications, she is the author of the health chapters in the Bank's flagship reports *eTransform Africa: The Transformational Use of Information and Communication Technologies in Africa* (2012); *Repositioning Nutrition as Central to Development* (2006); *Scaling Up Nutrition: What Will It Cost?* (World Bank, 2009); and most recently, *An Investment Framework for Nutrition: Reaching the Global Targets for Stunting, Anemia, Breastfeeding and Wasting* (World Bank, 2016). Dr. Shekar serves as a commissioner for the forthcoming Lancet Commission on Obesity. She has been an adjunct professor at Tufts University and a guest speaker at several G8 preparatory events, including the G8 parliamentarians' conference in Canada. She serves on several advisory boards. She holds a Ph.D. in international nutrition, epidemiology and population studies from Cornell University and has consulted extensively, including with Johns Hopkins University Population Communications Services and Population Services International.